MW01621126

One Step at a Time

"Bill Kemsley is a living example of how attention to detail and a passion for sports can produce excellence in advanced age."

Erik Steinberg, Olympic Gold Medalist Ski Coach,
(Mens Downhill 1984)

....

"Backpacker Bill spells it out in his definitive guide to a healthy and long life. Whether hiking in the Rockies, the Kaibab Forest, the Vermillion Cliffs, or sitting around with a good cigar and much philosophizing and argument, Bill set me straight 49 years ago, for which I owe him my gratitude. For healthy and contented sunset years, you owe yourself this read by one of the elders of the tribe."

Justus Bauschinger
Founder of Class-5, Mountaineering Equipage

....

"Anyone who thru-hikes the Appalachian Trail end to end will be younger at heart, in better physical condition and will realize they are capable of doing anything in life."

Noel "The Singing Horseman" DeCavalcante
A.T. '89 and solo canoe of the Mississippi River '90

....

"Somehow, I don't know how it happened. But even I am an "elderly person." A senior citizen. And I owe my good health and stamina to a lifetime of walking, backpacking, and what Henry David Thoreau called, "sauntering." Please read Bill's book and take it to heart."

Ron Strickland
founder of the Pacific Northwest National Scenic Trail.

....

"I wouldn't be here today if it wasn't for the trail."

Nimblewill Nomad
oldest person to thru-hike the Appalachian Trail
at age 83 in 2021,
and second to hike all the National Scenic Trails and Historic Trails.

"A motivating book to get you off your chair and outside! A great gift idea of mom, dad, and yourself! Throughout this inspirational book Bill Kemsley shares his passion and wisdom as the senior statesman of the hiking community. It's everything you need to know and consider to enjoy the outdoors and stay healthy and active.

As a lifelong walker, hiker and book reader entering into geezer territory, I learned some new ideas I will incorporate into my daily walks and hikes. Excellent health tips, exercises and chock full of practical advice for the novice and experienced. If there's a recipe for staying healthy as we age, it's in this book! Power on and out the door with his considtent can-do message in every chapter!"

Paula Guerrein

Part of the Hikeanation family, a trip inspired by Bill Kemsley in 1980-81 to hike from the Pacific Ocean in San Francisco to the Atlantic in Delaware to promote the American Hiking Society.

"It's a truism that as we age, our abilities decline. Whether around the house or in the office, limitations emerge. Slowly. Over years. Of course, this includes hiking. But wait. There's something deceptive here. Maybe walking and hiking are like breathing, very much a part of just living. So, we set out on a hike we used to do and take the effort for granted.

"Two years ago. I took six grandchildren hiking in the French Alps. I was exhausted on the third day, but blamed it on an active second day. This summer I thought all I had to do was rest on day two. Mistake. Two years have gone by. Now 87, that wasn't enough, not even close.

"Bill Kemsley's new book is for those of us up in years who like to hike. Don't take the effort for granted. There is much to think about on this unassuming subject. Start by getting Bill's book!"

Jim Kern
founder with Bill Kemsley of the American Hiking Society
founder of the Florida National Scenic Trail,
Big City Mountaineers,
Hiking Trails for America,
and friend of Bill's for a half century.

One Step at a Time

A Geezer's Guide
to Living a Long and Healthy Life
Through Hiking

By William Kemsley Jr.

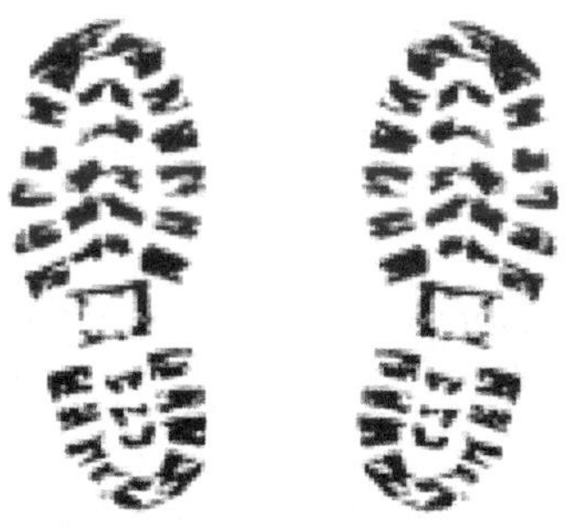

An
Appalachian Trail Museum
Publication

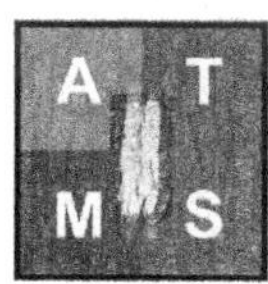

Published by The Appalachian Trail Museum

1120 Pine Grove Road

Gardners, Pa. 17324

www.atmuseum.org

Printed in the United States

First Edition

Cover design and book layout by Alan Strackeljahn

Editing by George Blackburn

ISBN 978-0-9912215-4-7

This book is dedicated to my good friend, Erik Steinberg, who coached me back from a severely crippling sciatica condition to a fine hiking form for my age. Without Erik's patient concern, I absolutely wouldn't be out hiking the trails today. Thanks to Erik, there's sure to be other geezers who will profit from his tips that I've tried to humbly pass on in this book.

Pick & Choose

A Good Way to Enjoy This Book
(Just a Suggestion)

I wrote this book on the assumption that most readers would want to take it bit by bit as their interests shift. Rather than read it straight through, it might be a lot more useful to pick and choose your way in it following your momentary interests, a few pages here and there, now and then.

On that assumption, I've repeated quite a few cardinal bits of advice so that you wouldn't miss them as you do your picking and choosing.

Take a Hike – Live Longer

Table of Contents

PREFACE

Are We Living on the Edge of an Aging Revolution?

When Roger Dubin put out a request for stories of geezers who believed their longevity was due to hiking, the response was overwhelming. He had to turn down stories of hikers in their sixties and seventies who were way too young for the article he was writing on "Longevity Through Hiking." (See: *https://naturalawakeningsli.com/longevity-through-hiking*)

Boomers Are Becoming Geezers

Boomers are now in their seventies. Many are hiking, causing *Outside* magazine editor, Gloria Liu, to refer to them as a major part of a comeback in recreational walking. (See: *https://www.outsideonline.com/2410054/gloria-liu*)

These geezers might even live ten years longer according to Harvard University studies. That is, if they also have four other healthy habits. They don't smoke, drink no more than six ounces of alcohol at a time, have an appropriate weight for their age, and mostly eat healthy foods.
(See: *https://news.harvard.edu/gazette/story/2018/04/5-healthy-habits*)

A Boom in Books and Articles on Hiking to Live Longer

There is a spate of articles and books about this phenomenon which give examples of geezers extending their lives through hiking. Try Googling "Hiking for Longevity." You might be surprised! There are plenty like Life-Span's. (See: *https://www.lifespan.org/lifespan-living/take-hike*)
And Intertwine's. (See: *https://www.theintertwine.org/outside-voice/live-longer-take-hike*)

But Don't Miss Hiking to Live to 100

The best I've found is a super article by Irena Macri in London's *Balance Festival* Journal for August 2016. She claims that if you ask centenarians what's the secret of their longevity, 56 percent of them worldwide will tell you that taking a hike at least once a week is an important part of it.

Macri is talking about getting started hiking from scratch and working your way all the way up to long treks to places like my favorite, the *Tour Du Mont Blanc*, a multi-day hike circling Mont Blanc through France, Italy and Switzerland. She recommends plenty of the more exotic treks, like the *Camino de Santiago* from France into northern Spain and the Everest Base Camp!
Okaaay! Check out her article at *https://www.balance-festival.com/Journal/August-2016/Natural-Anti-Ageing-with-Hiking*

Introduction

Bill Kemsley loves to hike. He's been spending time in the outdoors all his life. And for most of his life, *Backpacker Bill* has been encouraging others to hike and making it easier for them to do so.

At 93, he still loves to do a mile or so daily on the trails. And he wants others to enjoy hiking, as well. He wants to let you in on his secrets. With this book, he shows you how to have a longer, healthier and happier life.

When Bill got out of the Navy at the end of World War II, there were only two long-distance trails in the U.S. and far fewer hikers. A friend of mine, Dick Hudson, hiked the Appalachian Trail over a four-year period, from 1966 to 1970. Dick could remember every single hiker he met along the A.T. during those four years because there were so few hikers. Nowadays, it's generally impossible to remember all the hikers you meet in a single day on the A.T.

About that same time and in that same area where Dick lived, the lower Hudson River Valley, Bill encountered a huge increase in the number of hikers in the new generation on the trails. They weren't accustomed to trail etiquette. They were leaving a great deal of trash along the trails and were un-wise to the ways of the woods.

Elizabeth Levers of the New York-New Jersey Trail Conference noticed the same thing and started a Litter Day that has continued to be a major project of the Trail Conference and it has also garnered national attention.

Bill had a different idea. He started *Backpacker* Magazine in 1973. This was a few years after the first Earth Day and the first stirrings of backpacking becoming a more popular sport. 1973 was the first big year for long distance hikers on the A.T. and Bill poured gasoline on the flames. Before *Backpacker* was founded, fewer than 50 people had hiked the whole Appalachian Trail. Today, that many people and more finish the trail on a single beautiful autumn day on Mt. Katahdin in Maine.

A few years later, Bill got together with a couple of friends, Jim Kern and Paul Pritchard, to form the American Hiking Society to be the voice of hikers at the national level. With those same friends, Bill testified before Congress about the need for Federal help in building and protecting a national network of long trails.

These efforts succeeded far beyond the dreams of these pioneers. The National Trail System has grown from two National Scenic Trails in the late 1960s to eleven today. In addition, there are 19 National Historic Trails and thousands of National Recreation Trails. The mileage of trails on Federal lands has more than doubled and the trails are in much better shape. In the 1960s, most of these trails were barely hikeable. Today it is easy to get information on the trails and most are easy to follow. The problem today is finding a parking spot at trailheads anywhere in the U.S. and finding spots on the trails where they are not crowded.

More than just about anyone else, Bill Kemsley has played a key role in this revolution. And now he wants to extend this movement. He's not just promoting backpacking and hiking among young people. He's urging oldsters to lace up their boots and get out on the trail. If they do, Bill believes that they will get more joy out of life, live longer and healthier.

Who's to say Bill isn't on to something?

A few years ago, my wife, Frieda, and I joined Bill on a day hike in the pine covered mountains near his home in Taos, New Mexico. It is impossible to join Bill on a day hike and not feel the joy of the woods. We encountered several small groups of hikers as we wandered toward a creek. All got to sample a smile and a little conversation with Bill and left the woods a little happier.

Bill has a simple formula for spreading this joy even when you are tired, the weather is not optimal and the couch is calling. Give it a try. By the end of these few pages, I'll be surprised if you aren't ready to slip into your shoes, put your cares on the back burner and head for the woods and be glad you did.

Larry Luxenberg

Founder, Appalachian Trail Museum, and A.T. Thru-hiker in 1980

New City, N.Y., August 13, 2021

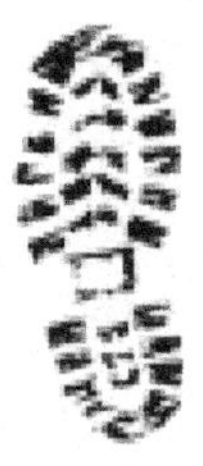

Chapter 1

Why Hike?

There are so many reasons why hiking is great for your health and will make you feel good, as well.

So please, whatever shape you're in, keep reading. You may be surprised. Regardless of your physical condition, if you can walk across a room, you can most likely get into hiking. In fact, it's best if you follow the advice of the good old geezer who founded the Sierra Club, John Muir. He said: "People ought to saunter, not hike . . ."

I have been hiking (or sauntering, per Muir) all of my life, and am still hiking on into my nineties. Most of my hiking these days actually is sauntering on very easy paths in the woods. Lately, it always seems as if I am "recovering" from one thing or another with my feet, legs or hips. I'm mentioning this now for encouragement, as a sort of 'if-he-can-do-it-I-can-do-it, too' way of urging you on.

Here Are Nine Good Reasons Why You Too Can Enjoy Hiking

1. *The first is foremost.* The joy of hiking helps get your butt out the door even on chilly days when you feel that the fireplace is more appealing.
2. *It's easy to hike no matter your physical condition.*
3. *It's good for your heart and your health.*
4. *You can walk when you cannot hike.* You can walk virtually any place you happen to be whether city or country, near a trail or only a sidewalk.
5. *The only equipment you need is a comfortable pair of shoes.* When you begin to hike a rougher trail, a pair of sneakers suffices. However, using trekking poles to prevent falling is a great bit of equipment worth the price.

6. *You do not need a partner*. You can hike alone providing you use common sense to let someone know where you are going and hike on a busy trail where there are plenty of other hikers who can help should you get into trouble.
7. *It relieves your mind of useless worries*. Hiking makes it difficult, if not impossible, to keep your mind on things that trouble you back home while you are out on a trail.
8. *It is a good place to be close to God*. Next to cathedrals and scripture it's compelling for the reverence you'll feel while in the woods.
9. *It's easy to meditate while hiking*. Later in the book I'll give you some tips for easy trail meditations.

Our Days Are Numbered. I know my end is near. And I'm getting wobblier by the day. I've had a series of health issues, one after another in the past couple of years. For I'm getting into what you might say is a more "limited" physical condition. Still, I'll be darned if I want to become so limited I can't take my hikes, even if they are just around the corridors of a hospital. So as I say, keep on hiking the best way possible. That is, if you want to enjoy your last few years as much as I'm enjoying mine.

At whatever age and condition, you never know what is going to happen in the next fifteen minutes!

Sure, I'm being a bit over the top, but these beliefs are an integral part of my life. I believe my walking and hiking are the major things that keep me going.

I hope I can persuade you to enjoy your life as I'm enjoying mine.

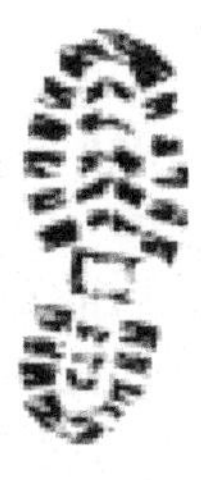

Chapter 2

How to Get Started Hiking If You've Never Hiked Before: GO FOREST BATHING

Forest Bathing is not hiking — Of course. But, it may be the easiest, healthiest and most laid-back way of taking your first slow saunter in the woods. Actually, you don't even need to *walk* anywhere to get started. You can go *forest bathing* by simply sitting quietly on a bench among trees.

You might even just spend ten minutes in a quiet nook of New York City's Central Park. As long as it's away from the Big Apple's noise, it can be "medical therapy for urban-frayed nerves," as one journalist puts it.

If you are approaching retirement and have never spent any time on a hiking trail, Forest Bathing could be something more congenial for starters than taking your first hike on a rugged mountain trail. The Japanese began forest bathing as a gentle way to become better acquainted with the trees and streams of the forests. They call it *Shinrin-yoku.* And doctors are prescribing a slow walk in the woods to heal many of the illnesses of aging – hypertension, depression, heart disease.

According to Doctor Qing Li, a leading proponent of the medical benefits of forest bathing and founder of the Japanese Society for Forest Medicine, "it reduces stress, anxiety, depression, and anger. And it strengthens the immune system; improves cardiovascular and metabolic health; and boosts overall well-being." Doctor Li is author of *Forest Bathing*, a popular, authoritative book. It might be the perfect way of familiarizing yourself with the woods before striding off overly confident on your first hike.

American doctors are following the Japanese by urging their patients to spend some time in the woods as an antidote to anxieties, depression and other health issues. Even if you only try forest bathing, but never take a hike, you will improve your well-being from just a few visits to the woodlands. It's a win for your health.

Forest Bathers Avoid Doing Anything Strenuous.

You can follow their example. Go into the woods. Spend from ten minutes to an hour or so, just moseying about and taking notice of the woodlands around you. It's restful just being in the woods away from your television, computer and cell-phone. Resting in the woods allows your body to throttle down and heal the city's stresses.

Your body will absorb an emission of a subtle substance from the trees called *phytoncides*, which carry the trees' medicinal effect. Forest bathing is so simple and so easy. It seems the perfect cure-all for the stress Americans suffer today from city-living noise, cell-phones, computers, television and other digital devices.

Health Benefits of Forest Bathing

When we suffer from stress it takes a toll on our bodies' defensive health capabilities. Unchecked stress can lead to hypertension, depression, obesity and heart disease. Japanese studies show that forest bathing reduces your cortisol levels, which in turn, slows your heart rate, lowers your blood pressure, and stimulates your immune system. Cortisol is an unhealthy substance generated in part by stress. According to still other studies, people actually *feel* better and *think* better when they spend time in the woods. All it takes is becoming still, ridding all thoughts from your mind and allowing yourself to touch and feel the leaves and rough bark of the trees. And smell the faint scent of the forest moisture shortly after it rains.

I know, it seems way too simple, getting such health benefits from just going into the woods, turning off your phone, freeing yourself of all your worries and *allowing* yourself to listen, see, smell, feel and even taste the forests' subtle sensations. There are professionally trained guides who can lead you through the basics of forest bathing. They will take you on a visit to the woods to show you how to best experience the sensuality of the forest.

Guides, for example, will take you either in a group, or privately, through a series of easy practices to experience the forest — the texture of leaves and tree bark, hear bird songs, see the sun's rays filtering down through the trees and feel its soft warmth on the bare skin of your face and hands.

Do-It-Yourself Forest Bathing

Realizing though, that many of us don't live near a professional guide service, National Public Radio has published a set of instructions on how to take a do-it-yourself forest bath.
Here is an outline of the NPR suggestions.

1. Find the right place – like a woodland park away from the city's hustle and bustle, with plenty of trees and fewer people.
2. Choose a time and duration that's right for you – a time when you can get away from your everyday activities. And whenever you can, feel free to sit quietly for ten to fifteen minutes. Longer if possible.
3. Take only what's necessary with you – a bottle of drinking water, warm, comfortable clothing.
4. Turn off your phone.
5. Go slowly – and let your senses experience what's around you.
6. Notice small things – feel the warmth of the sun on your face, hear the wind in the trees, feel the breezes on the bare skin of your face and hands.
7. Observe – notice the plants growing on the forest floor, the patterns in leaves, tree bark, and stones.

Forest bathing is an excellent way to start becoming familiar with the woods. Don't hesitate about going by yourself, if guides aren't possible; but whichever way, get out there. Allow yourself to simply be there. Meditate if you like. Take time to appreciate your surroundings. Listen for the twittering of birds and the breezes rustling leaves. Breathe in the fresh, fragrant air. Soak in sights and textures of the forest floor. Touch and feel the soft, green moss and the cool smooth stone surfaces. Let the stillness influence your state of mind. Forget the constant motion of the city.

Forest bathing is a spiritual cleansing of the mind as taking a bath cleanses the body. If you are a geezer who's been mostly house-and-workplace-bound for too long, it would be splendid if you gave forest bathing a shot. Begin with walking to a quiet place in a wooded park, stop and rest, taking your time in a "forest bath" for awhile, then finish your walk back out. This provides an easy beginning from which to build up your *feel* for the woodlands and may spur you to try some trail *sauntering*.

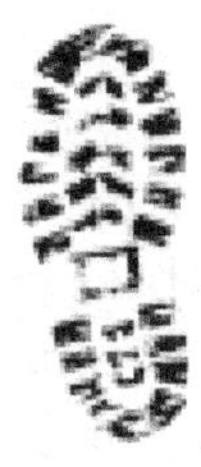

Chapter 3

How to Get Started Hiking Again

If you are an experienced hiker, away from the trail for a few years, or if you are new to the trail and never hiked before, my advice is pretty much the same. A good beginning might be to join a walking or hiking group at a YMCA or local health club in your area. Check to see if your insurance company offers Silver Sneakers, some of which have walking offerings. It's a great benefit offered by many companies.

Then, please, if you are about to head out on an extended hike with friends, I'd strongly urge 'an ounce of prevention.' *Get permission from your doctor to take the hike.* And, of course, do everything possible to get into shape before shouldering your pack. If your doctor gives you an okay, I next advise finding the maximum heart rate for your age and physical condition. I cover this at the end of this chapter and in more detail in Chapter 12, *Hiking with a Heart Condition*.

As we age, we tend to rely too heavily on our memories of old times when we used to hike with considerable ease. This could be deadly to an experienced hiker who jumps back into strenuous hiking after years of little to no physical exercise.

It sounds silly, of course. You'd be surprised, though, at how many geezers turn sixty, give in to this temptation and end up in the ER right off a trail they easily hiked at thirty. To determine your safe heart rate, take an easy walk while monitoring your heart rate. Whenever your breathing becomes at all noticeable, slow your pace to its prescribed limits.

Start slowly as if you're in a training camp.

Do all you can to succeed.

So Let's Go Hiking

Hiking is the best exercise for prolonged good physical health. I'm in my nineties and still hiking. You shouldn't be surprised that I believe my hiking regimen got me through heart issues as well as other life-threatening illnesses – extending my active life into my nineties. I don't see why you too can't have the same results.

I hope I can convince you to accept your aging and truly enjoy the years you still have coming. You too, with an "easy-does-it" hiking program, might have a healthier, safer, longer and far more exciting life than you've ever imagined.

Start by taking short, easy walks. Take one every day. Be easy on yourself from the first walk, so that you don't easily quit. Gradually increase your time on the trail, watching that you do not exceed your safe heart rate. Increase your walking distance a little each day until you reach an optimum, enjoyable daily hiking routine.

You should soon actually look forward to taking your hikes.

Create a Routine

Work on your attitude from the beginning. You are getting older. *Accept it*. Go about this whole program knowing you are a geezer. Stick to the three 'S's. Go Slowly, Sensibly and Steadily.

While you will likely benefit from a more strenuous hike occasionally, it gets riskier as you age. Sudden, excessive exertion can easily cause a heart attack, and heart attacks are the leading cause of death among geezers. Worse still, in my opinion, is the threat of a stroke. A stroke could paralyze you and thus prevent you from walking, never mind hiking, for the rest of your life. I'd personally like to avoid the wheelchair if at all possible.

The Good News

You do not need to be "in shape" to get started. Being out of shape might make it easier for you to stick to a slower, gradual walking routine. Also, you're not so likely to have unattainable goals. It took me a few years to realize I was no longer going to be hiking my old mountain trails. There have been a few summers I envisioned climbing a few peaks I'd long had my eyes on. Admittedly, I ended those summers sadly disappointed. But I got over it. And you, too, can do that. Expect this. It is a resistance that you too can muddle through. You may be surprised at what acceptance of your aging can do for you. Give it a little time. You too may be able to find the happiness I've found in "slowing down" as the clock ticks.

Follow Your Inner Clock

If you can walk, you are most likely in good enough shape to hike, and even if you are already in good shape and want to get into hiking as a geezer, give it a chance. So my second proviso: Don't try to walk at a faster pace or longer distances than is prudent for your age and physical condition. Instead, let consistency become your goal. Resolve to take a walk every day, and don't let it die like a New Year's resolution! Some coaches suggest aerobics, but they are used to training younger guys, and may not be as savvy about our aging. I say instead, ***do not*** put aerobics into your thinking. There will be time enough for you to move on up from walking into hiking where heavy breathing will come naturally. Being consistent is best achieved by taking it easy. So enjoy walking from the beginning. If you make it arduous, you are bound to fail. So *easy does it*. Assure yourself you'll do it.

Why Taking It Easy Will Save Your Life

Start with only a fifteen-minute walk a day. If I could do it, so can you.

Here's my story. When I was in my sixties, I had a heart attack requiring open-heart surgery. Immediately after surgery, the cardiologist had me up and walking. As I went home from the hospital, he made me promise I'd walk just fifteen minutes *every* day. I did.

That was thirty years ago. And I am still walking every day. I've had three painful back and leg issues in the past few years that made it impossible for me to walk across a room. Each time, though, I followed the advice the heart surgeon had given me after my surgery. And soon I was out and walking fifteen minutes every day. There's a psychological component to fifteen-minute walks. It's easier to get out and walk at times when you least want to. You develop the 'what the heck; why not?' attitude, knowing, 'It's *only* fifteen minutes!'

Soon I began walking twenty-minutes a day. Shortly after that, I moved up a notch to twenty-five minutes a day. Then thirty. Then I moved up to an easy hiking trail. And so on, until I was doing good, strenuous hikes each day.

When I absolutely didn't want to hike, I dropped back to my fifteen-minute walk. But I walked. It helped me avoid the "New Year's resolution syndrome." It just takes steadiness and time. If you do, God forbid, miss even the fifteen-minute walk, it's easier to get started again. Forgive yourself and take the first opportunity to start over again. Just think, "It's only fifteen-minutes." And make it work. Start over. It's okay. You're going for saving your life and staying in shape.

Don't give up.

It's only fifteen minutes!

Easy Does It Hiking

Don't rush it. *The most important part of your walking is to walk every day*. And only after a few weeks or months of daily walking, add gentle hiking trails to your walks. You will know when the time has come.

I've found that I still mix into my daily routine an occasional "hike" on a packed gravel path in the woods. It is a one-mile loop, with an almost unnoticeable elevation change along the way. It is just like a walk in the park back in the city. But it gives me a break; especially on those days when I don't feel like a hike.

The American Heart Association assures us that a mere twenty-five-minute walk daily substantially reduces your risk of stroke and heart attack. I cannot emphasize it enough. Take it easy. No matter how good your physical condition; if you aren't already hiking on a regular basis, start with just an easy fifteen-minute daily walk. You are far more likely to stick to it, if you do an easy hike *every* day. I'm emphasizing the word *every.* That's the key to overcoming that unexpected resistance when you do not feel like hiking.

You'll feel good about yourself for having won – even if it is just for a fifteen-minute walk. And when you least wanted to do it. Eventually, after beating your resistances, you'll move your daily walk up a notch, say to a *thirty*-minute walk six days a week with a day off. *But, beware of over-ambitious thinking!*

Don't Try to Prove Anything

While it can be tempting at times to prove how much you can do despite your senior years, fifteen minutes a day is enough. It is easy to take out of your busiest day, even if you have to take your walk with a flashlight late in the evening. Not even *speed* walking. Just walk. Am I repeating myself? That's the point, because it sounds all too easy sitting at home reading about it. You are playing with your life. Especially the older you get. You are gambling with the quality of life ahead of you.

How to Progress from Walking to Hiking

You are ready for hiking once you are walking about thirty minutes a day. Even earlier for hiking easy trails. I still hike daily on a trail that is more a smooth path through the woods than a hiking trail. And it has very little difference in elevation in its one-mile circle. I also switch to hiking a couple of miles on more difficult trails about once or twice a week.

You're actually ready, though, when you say you are. Obviously, you'll want to start on easier trails. Go for it, but with moderation. Remember: the biggest bug-a-boo for geezers are falls and heart attacks.

Don't become a dead hero. Use your God-given common sense. Easy does it.

How to Avoid Falling While Hiking.

First off, use hiking poles. It's a good way to reduce the chances of taking a fall, which is increased among those of us who hike. And that is even higher than it is among all seniors. One out of every four geezers over 65 will take a fall *every* year. And these falls are the leading cause of fatal injuries among us seniors. Please, don't become a statistic. Work at avoiding falls. Geezers tend to develop poor posture as we age. And this makes us even more prone to falls. Learn how to work on your posture, even while hiking. (See Chapter 13 *Correct Your Posture While Hiking*)

How to Avoid Heart Issues While Walking

As you begin your walking routine, try to develop the habit of checking your heart rate from time to time. Check especially whenever you notice your breathing becoming noticeably labored. Here's how. Find out what your maximum heart rate is for your age. Do this before you even set foot outdoors. It's an easy calculation. Deduct your age from the number 220. That gives you the maximum safe heart rate for people your age. If you are 60, for example, then 220 minus 60 is 160. That is your maximum heart rate.

Maximum Heart Rate for Your First Walks

Regardless of your physical condition, start your routine slowly. For your first walking, be sure your heart does not exceed half your maximum heart rate. If you are 60, then half your maximum heart rate of 160 is 80. So check your heart rate as your breathing becomes noticeable. If it is above 80, stop, rest and wait for it to return to 80 before you begin walking again.

In time, as you become comfortable while walking, allow your tolerable heart rate to move up gradually, but not more than what it is when your breathing becomes labored. Eventually, as you build your endurance, you may move your tolerable heart rate up to about three-quarters of your maximum. For a 60-year-old that would be seventy-five percent of 160, making it 120. No more than this without your doctor's consent. (I go into greater detail in *Chapter 12 – Hiking with a Heart Condition.)*

Chapter 4

Getting the Get Up and Go — When You Least Want To

Do yourself a life-saving favor. Have a purpose for your life. Those who do have a purpose to live, regardless of their age, have a seventy-seven percent better chance of *avoiding death from all causes,* according to studies at Mount Sinai St. Luke's Medical Center. How about living longer by making hiking a purpose for your life. All that's necessary is telling yourself, "Hiking is a good *purpose* to live." And remind yourself of it as often as possible.

How to Activate Your Purpose

I suspect you are reading this book because you'd like to form a hiking habit. It's easy to *want* to form a habit. But habits we'd like to have don't usually turn into real habits. W*anting* a hiking habit if you've only hiked a few times will probably sound formidable! And especially daunting if you've never ever hiked. The idea of turning it into a life's purpose by just telling yourself you'd like it, probably sounds even zanier. Not to worry! It may actually be easier than you think. Stick with me.

The Power of Bite-size Thinking

Reading a book looks formidable, too. But, you have to read it *one-page-at-a-time*, which makes it far less intimidating to start reading it. Why not do the same with forming a hiking purpose? How about building a hiking habit in bite-size-pieces.

The first bite-size step in taking a hike is putting on your hiking shoes. That's simple enough. And not daunting. So, go ahead. Start your daily hiking habit, as silly as it sounds, by just putting on your hiking shoes. Honestly, as dumb as this sounds, it can increase your chances immeasurably of forming a daily hiking habit.

So get started – by taking your first bite-size step. Sit down, pull on a hiking shoe and lace it up. Then the next. All the time, allow the thought to run through your mind, 'If I don't want to go hiking when I get the shoes on, then I won't.' No further thoughts about it. Just do it. Then, just as deliberately, unlace your hiking shoes, one at a time, telling yourself, "I am not going hiking today. And that's okay." And don't go. Be sure to tell yourself, "It's okay."

This first little task has to be so easy that you'll actually do it every day, whether you want to take a hike or not. On those days you don't feel like it, it will be a relief to tell yourself, "No, I'm not going hiking today." Then, on these days, turn around, sit down, unlace your hiking shoes, take them off and do not go hiking. If this sounds as if I'm suggesting that you develop a bad habit, of *not* going hiking, think twice. It actually is the beginning of forming a habit.

How to Take Charge of Yourself

The benefit of forming this simple bite-size habit is in taking charge of yourself. To hike when you want to and not feel guilty if you don't. I really am urging you to take this small step as a measure *in taking control of yourself*. This time it is about forming a hiking habit. But the same bite-size formation of habits can be applied for any other self-improvement you'd like. So, show yourself that – "*From now on I'm the boss.*" Tell yourself, *"I'll not allow an old habit to run my life another day."*

This little trick will make a significant difference in your life. Try it today. Put on your hiking shoes. And then take them off. See how that feels. Do this every day for two weeks, without taking a hike. Put on your hiking shoes; and take them off. Then, when the day comes that you cannot resist taking a short stroll on a trail, then go for it. But do not yet make a commitment to take another.

There are two major resistances to forming a hiking habit:

1. Taking the first step on the trail.
2. Keeping on taking hikes when you least want to.

With this practice, you're building a bit-by-bit process, an easy way of working on the first of these resistances.

How to Go for a Hike Regardless of How You Feel

Begin by allowing yourself the freedom of taking a hike whenever you want. And *not* taking one when you don't feel like it. Do this as long as it takes to form a habit of putting on your hiking shoes, so strong that you daren't miss a single day. Once you have actually formed a rock solid habit, then move up a step. Add another bite-size habit. Go to your door with your boots on and return to your chair, unlace your shoes and take them off. Feel free during this period to go for a hike if you have a burning desire to get to trekking. But, at this point, it's important not to force yourself to go if you don't feel like it. Take your time. You are dealing with something very precious — your life! Work on this process as if you were going to the office or plant where you earned a living. Think of it as your most important task each day. *Saving your life ought to be a worthy purpose!* So it's worth every bit of the effort.

My Hiking Purpose In Life

My own purpose is to do whatever I possibly can to keep on my feet 'til I die. I want desperately to avoid ending up in a wheelchair. And so far, so good! It keeps me going for at least a short, easy hike every day. And a half hour a day of my stretch exercises. I take a hike and do my stretch exercises, whether I feel like it or not. I built these habits in bits and pieces. The same as I'm suggesting you to do it.
I am in charge of myself. And I want to keep it that way. I formed my habits in as silly a way as I'm urging you to do it. I'm in my nineties and still on my feet, and out on a trail every day!

If you are consistent and actually do lace up your hiking shoes every day, even when you least want to hike, you'll be surprised at the results. You'll actually be well on your way to a new habit. Oh, above all, remind yourself during this entire process that you are putting purpose into your life for your physical well-being. The inertia of getting ready to go will eventually overcome your lethargy, get you up and out the door and hiking. Newton's First Law of Motion that "Things in motion tend to stay in motion" will eventually prevail.

Next, use the same bite-size strategy for other segments of your hikes. You don't have to be the least bit athletic to get out the door and take a few steps on a walk. Always give yourself short, easily achievable goals. Say five to ten minute walks at the early part of your self-training. Stick to whatever goal you set. So be easy on yourself. Almost childishly easy. When you walk that short distance goal, and you feel up to it, you may want to walk further. That's fine, go ahead and walk on, but with a new proviso. You will allow yourself to turn back at any time you feel like it. And tell yourself, "It's okay to turn back." And not to feel guilty about it.

If you simply do these little exercises, you will have begun a healthy hiking habit.

How Best to Use Bite-Size Objectives

Have a large purpose in life. But, use small, bite-size targets to move toward it. Give yourself permission to regularly achieve smaller goals. Fulfill each small target. And nothing more - until it becomes a habit.

I found that when I still felt sluggish, even after I'd laced up my hiking shoes, that was it. I put them away for the day, but the time came when I wanted to push myself a little. So, I'd set myself another small goal that I knew I could easily achieve. It might be just getting up and going to the door. And when I'd be at the door, I'd keep my promise to myself. And go back, sit down, unlace my hiking shoes, take them off. And I don't hike that day! Today, of course, these episodes are rare. However, when I was recovering from my last sciatic episode, I had to begin with these small achievements, getting to the door and no further because of the pain. With each bite-size step of the process, I eventually got to the trailhead and no further. I well recall how I couldn't even get out of the car at the trailhead at first, never mind think of hiking. It was okay, for that was my bite-size goal.

In a few days I was able to get out to the trailhead, each time giving myself my word of honor that I would turn back if I felt like it. Next goal was to get to the first trail junction. Then to the trail sign at the *Anasazi Kiva*. Or a hundred paces beyond that. And with each new goal, I set the same parameters. Stop and go no farther until I knew for sure I could get to the next target, without turning back. If at any step along the way my pain hadn't improved, I didn't go any farther.

But, reading about it and thinking you'll do it leaves out something. It still requires action. Why not try it? Right now? See if you can't start with one tiny step today. I mean, set this book down and go put on your hiking shoes. Then leave it at that. Unlace your shoes and take them off. Come back to the book and resolve to simply do it every day, including those dark and gloomy days ahead. But just do it for two weeks as a start on a hiking habit.

And when you start to hike, break the hike down, too, into bite-size pieces, adding one small bite, after another, until you've reached your goal for a day. At whatever point in a hike you reach each day, you *must, absolutely must*, stick to small objectives. Once you reach that objective, then turn back if you feel like it. Only go on if you have a burning desire for more hiking. You ought not have any "musts." Not even must reach your target. It's just an idea you've set out to achieve. There's nothing sacred about it. Remember, it's about you talking charge of your life.

If, for instance, you are feeling real bullish one day and set an ideal goal for your daily hikes, but a day or two later find just thinking about hiking is exhausting, there is nothing wrong with adjusting your sights down a peg or two. What is defeating, is to give up and not set another shorter goal. I know. I've done exactly that sort of goal adjustment. Many times!

YOU can take charge of YOUR LIFE!

You can do it if you . . . *Take charge of it in bite-size pieces*.

I've used this dumbed-down goal-setting technique to get back into hiking when I thought it impossible.

I've applied this technique to many other purposes in my life as well, to raise a family, to write books - even to start-up a magazine. Even to just get through a tough day.

If it seems like I'm repeating myself, *I am*. It is a system that works. Don't belittle it. Believe me, starting a magazine from scratch is nothing to sneeze at. Sending out the first issue of *Backpacker* magazine was the scariest thing I ever did. When magazine start-ups were costing several million dollars, I don't think I could have scraped together more than a few thousand dollars beyond the operating funds I needed to run my very small business. Yet I had a wife and six small children who depended upon my weekly paycheck. It was no time for slip-ups! It took three years of itty bitty goals, testing my way, step by step, before I dared to press the "Go" button and actually send out that first issue to people who subscribed to my commitment to send each of them further issues.

I'll usually feel a little better at each one of the small points I see ahead of me, willing to go a bit farther and then a bit farther than that, eventually completing a full-blown accomplishment. Even to taking a short hike on a day I feel shitty!

The trick is that at each ridiculously small goal, I say something like this to myself, "Okay, I've come this far. If I go to the next goal, which might be just driving to the trailhead or hiking to the next trail junction, and I don't feel like even getting out of my truck, I don't. I'll allow myself to turn around, come back home and not hike at all." Usually, though, I hope that by then Newton's *first* law of motion will be at work and "The thing, *Me*, in motion will stay in motion. And, *I*, will take the hike."

Eventually, after you've been hiking regularly, your feet won't let you stay away from the trail. It's sort of like the fairy tale movie, *The Red Shoes*. Leading lady, ballerina Moira Shearer, becomes victim of her 'red shoes' that compel her to keep on dancing — on and on and on and on. She cannot stop dancing. For the compulsive pull of those damned red shoes! Eventually Shearer's red shoes drag her along to her demise! This may sound way too simple-minded for someone as intelligent as you. Give yourself a break. Allow yourself to be as simple-minded as it takes to make your New Year's Resolutions come true. Dumber geezers than you have gone on to win world championships through these training techniques. So, it might be time to give it a shot. It could well mean the well-being of the last decades of your earthly life.

Patience!

Get used to walking before you go hiking. Your regularity and consistency are what count. Make your aim a daily walk or hike. Do not be concerned about how far or how fast you can or ought to hike. Comparing your walking to better hikers, even to what you did back in your twenties - dooms you to failure. Make your habit of hiking the joy of the outdoors rather than how far you can go or how fast.

Set Achievable Hiking Goals

Make your small incremental goals achievable. But don't be too rigid about adhering to them. Otherwise it can lead to failure of your whole intention. I suggest the larger goal of *daily* hiking. It's more likely you'll achieve a daily goal than trying to hike two or three times a week. For good reason. It's easier to remember to do something every time the sun comes up, than trying to remember which days of the week you had planned to hike. And there's less mañana temptation, the "I'll put off my hike until tomorrow." At least it has been for me. It just seems much, much easier for me to establish a rhythm of daily hiking, than for occasional hikes. Then too, regularity guarantees the most enjoyment. Once you are out the door and on your walk, your feet will tell you how far and how long to go. Don't become too rigid. Just follow them.

Easy Does It

Be patient with yourself. When I was recovering from serious surgery, for instance, I was supposed to walk fifteen minutes a day, every day. So that became my daily target. But as I've said, I'll give myself permission to turn back, even if I haven't gone out the door yet. On such days it is natural that I'd feel like a failure later on for not having walked. I've had to train my head to understand it is all right if I turn back and don't hike for the day. And not to feel guilty about it! That was regardless of how often I turned back. It was okay. And no guilt about it. That was my agreement with myself. And I stuck to it.

It was useful to remind myself of an old marksman's adage "You don't learn how to hit the bulls-eye by hitting the bulls-eye." It would almost immediately turn the idea of failure into one of success. I'd just substitute the word habit for bulls-eye when I'd bring the adage to mind. I'd remind myself that having the habit does not form a habit. Thus, like missing the bulls-eye again and again, my aim got nearer and nearer to my bulls-eye. I found that I was turning back fewer and fewer times – at the door, at the trailhead or at the next switchback along the trail – my hiking habit became more firmly entrenched.

Find Ways to Enjoy Hiking

Another motivational help is to find ways to make your hikes as enjoyable as possible. Probably the easiest way to make them enjoyable is to find your best hiking pace and stick to it. This will be one small way to help you look forward to getting out onto a trail.

Consider one of the most tiresome sides of younger hikers. It's annoying trying to adjust to their hiking pace. It took me a while to figure out how to deal with it. No matter who I'm hiking with, I stick to my pace. (Chapter 9 gives details on how to find your most comfortable hiking pace.)

Sticking to it, though, is challenging while hiking with others. I find the more I hike at my comfortable pace, the less I am bothered by "trying to keep up" to their faster pace. I don't try to keep up even with my wife and close friends. My wife, Joy, often hikes with me these days. She's a lot younger than me, so finds it difficult to slow her pace down to mine. My usual hike is on a trail that is a mile-long loop. So she'll lap me, leaving me to saunter along at my pace. And we'll meet back at the trailhead at the end of my hike. Both happy we've hiked another day.

Other Hikers On the Trail

Allow other hikers to pass you. Remind yourself that you are not twenty anymore. And you are out to enjoy your hiking.

I tell you all this as though it were easy. And it is easy for me *to write* about it. But it was difficult for me to work these things out while out on a trail with faster hikers. Practice, though, has enabled me to thoroughly enjoy hiking regardless of the pace of others on a hike. I remind myself over and over again, that what others may think about my hiking is of no concern to me. Not anymore! In fact, you will find that in time, people will actually admire you for your ability to enjoy yourself on a hike.

I Had a Comeuppance Recently

I had an attack of sciatica so severe that I could barely hobble across a room on crutches. At the onset, there were days when my legs and back hurt so much, I didn't want to *try* to walk across a room, even on crutches. But, my wife kept gently urging me *to try*. She'd say something like this: "Why not walk only as far as you feel you can." I would try it. Even on my worst days. I could usually make it across the room. On crutches at first. Then, after a few days, with hiking poles. Then, finally, with neither. My good friend, Erik, at that point, urged me to take a few steps out on a trail. We'd take the easiest trail possible – level, hard-packed surface with no rocks or roots to trip on. No matter how bad I felt, it was imperative that I walk *somewhere*. For whatever distance I could. It took me a little over three months to be back hiking at my usual pace again. Without pain.

I urge you to get started. But remember 'moderation in all things' – including hiking. Set a purpose. One that you really want to achieve. Break it up into bite-size pieces. Move toward it at your most comfortable pace.

Enjoy good health and longer life.

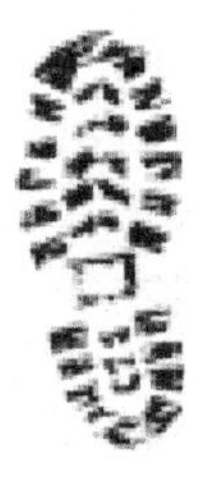

Chapter 5

Outfitting Your Clothing and Gear

If you are taking your first walk and have comfortable shoes you needn't read any farther in this chapter. All you need is the will to walk. So, instead of reading, take a fifteen-minute walk. And feel great at your accomplishment. You can read the rest of the chapter at any time.

If, on the other hand, you are ready to hike, but don't have good shoes, then continue reading. The good thing about hiking is that you probably already have all the clothing you need to get started. Any loose-fitting, casual clothes are good enough. And, any comfortable shoes are good enough to get started.

Take an easy hike, on an easy trail, in moderate weather, wearing whatever you can scrounge from your clothes closet.

See If You Like Hiking

If you do and your finances permit, then at your leisure, you can begin changing your attire into whatever you find to be more suitable for the trail. But do keep in mind *layering*. No need to worry, though. For if you forget, you will soon learn the need for it on your hikes.

What Is Proper Hiking Clothing?

You needn't feel at all self-conscious about the way you dress for a hike. In America we have no "hiking clothes," despite the abundant racks of fashionable clothing in sporting goods stores. I live in Taos, New Mexico, where probably a third of our population are hikers. And you'd never guess it from the clothing we wear on the trails.

Nonetheless, there are some basics that apply no matter how fashionable your clothing. To get started hiking, just dress sensibly. Better you begin your hike dressed too warmly, than not warmly enough. You can always take off a jacket, sweater or heavier shirt if you get too warm. But you can't put it on if you haven't brought it with you.

Protection Against Insects

Now, a bit about shorts and short-sleeve shirts. They are a no no. Mostly because of insects. But also sunburn. This is especially true at higher elevations where air is thinner making the sun's rays more intense. I always wear long sleeve shirts and long pants. And if I'll be hiking on a trail through higher grasses and brush, I tuck my pant legs into my socks to avoid ticks. I spray a good insect repellent especially about the openings of the cuffs of my sleeves and the bottom of the legs of my pants for protection against ticks. Almost everywhere in America ticks are prevalent and carry serious diseases like Lyme disease and Rocky Mountain spotted fever. So, I'm maybe paranoid, but I don't like to take even small chances. One of my daughters wasn't as concerned. She got Lyme disease and was never free of its symptoms for the rest of her life. You needn't fear hiking because of ticks. Just take the necessary precautions – long sleeves, long legged pants, tuck pant legs in socks and spray strong insect repellent at all openings of sleeves and pants.

Adjust to Weather by Layering

Wear thin layers of clothes, one atop the other. Instead of wearing one heavy sweater, for example, wear two thin shirts or a thin shirt and sweater, one atop the other. Common sense tells you that when you get warm, you can take off the top layer. Or when the temperature drops, add a shirt or sweater.

Outerwear

On cool mornings I wear a lightweight nylon jacket. It weighs only a few ounces. It's a bit water-resistant, making it handy to carry in my pack. After fifteen minutes or so I take it off to prevent myself from working up a sweat. On longer pack-off rest stops, I slip the jacket back on to keep from getting chilled. As I get ready to resume hiking, of course, I take the jacket off and put it in the top of my pack where it will be handy. I live in the Southwest high mesa desert country. We get less rain out here than where I lived back east. So, except during monsoon season, we're safe carrying just this bit of outer layer clothing. Back east I carried both a light jacket as well as rain gear on most hikes. Know your local weather conditions. Dress and carry extra clothing accordingly. When I hike three hours or more, I carry my rain parka instead of the jacket. It provides warmth and is far better rain protection. When you've decided you'll do more hiking, you'll want to visit a sporting goods store and gradually acquire synthetic clothing — pants, shirts and outer wear. Be sure to shop with knowledgeable clerks and seriously consider their advice.

Socks

Avoid cotton socks, just as you should avoid cotton clothing. Cotton holds moisture and cools your body rapidly. There are a great many brands of excellent hiking socks. My favorites are the inexpensive LL Bean Merino Wool Ragg socks. I've re-ordered them so many times that I've lost track. You might also consider wearing a thin pair of nylon socks beneath your wool socks. These will protect against blisters since they cling to your foot, while the outer socks move against the inside of the boot.

Hiking Boots

Your boot will be the most important item of equipment you will need. If you are ready to buy your first pair, you might want the low-cut boot. Not only is it less expensive, it is easiest to fit. And a good fit in a hiking boot is critical. Most good sporting-goods shops stock several brands of boots because manufacturers use different lasts to make them. And each brand of boot, therefore, fits differently. A knowledgeable sales person can tell you which brand will more likely be appropriate for your feet. Whether it has, for example, a wide or narrow heel, a high or low arch, and other particularities to be comfortable on your feet after a few miles on a trail. Do not lean too heavily on the boot brand or sales person in making your decision. You are the only one who knows how the boots feel on your feet. Do not let anyone persuade you differently! Hopefully, you're into hiking for the long haul. And a boot that irritates can become discouraging!

Finding Your Right Boot Fit. Your normal boot size is only a starting point. You'll want to have your foot size measured before buying your boots. Your feet expand a bit when hiking. Age too, can cause your feet to expand. I'm now wearing a half size bigger boot than when I was a few years ago. Then too, manufacturers' boot sizes often don't match up with street shoe sizes. Finally, you are the only judge of the comfort of the boots, even if it defies logic.

Seven Tests for a Perfect Boot Fit

Most hiking stores have a variety of socks for you to put on when trying on boots. But it is far better for fitting if you take along a pair of your own hiking socks. Have the sales person measure your feet while you are wearing socks. To get the best measurement, stand with all your weight on each foot while measuring. The Brannock foot scale is a good measure. Trust it. Your sales person will no doubt take you through other tests for a good fit.

1. First, you ought to try a few different brands, as well as different sizes.

As a rule of thumb, try on several brands and sizes of boots, narrowing them down to about three boot options you like most.

2. As soon as you have on a boot, kick your heel all the way into the back of it. Then lace up the boots as tightly as you can.
3. Squat into a knee bend or two to see if the heel slips up and down. If it slips more than about an eighth of an inch, try on another boot.
4. To test the correct width at the ball of the foot, have someone hold your foot firmly in place. Then try to rotate your foot. You should not be able to feel any movement while trying to rotate it. The object is to get enough toe wiggle-room. But not any rotation of the ball, which can cause blisters.
5. Being sure you have laced the boot tightly, now kick the toe of the boot to the floor. Try to kick your toes to the front of the boot. If the fit is right, your toes will not touch the toe of the boot.
6. Try on several sizes and brands of boots, regardless of price or looks.

7. Try on one boot of a pair on one foot. Then a boot of another pair on the other foot. Feel the difference of the two. Now, take off the less friendly boot and try on a different size or brand. And compare the fit of these two. Again, take off the lesser of the two. Replace it with a different size or brand. Now again remove the boot that is the less comfortable of these two. And so on, until you find the boot model and size that fits best. Then put on the other boot of this pair and walk around the store a while to see how that feels. If you want to develop a hiking habit, it is imperative that your boots fit properly.

My wife recently bought a pair of boots mainly because they were great looking, and partly because of an attractive mark down price. After just one hike she was enormously disappointed.

Fortunately, the store where she bought them, REI, was customer-friendly and exchanged them for another pair that fit properly, though they cost twice as much. Now she's so pleased with them, she hates to take them off after our hikes.

Waterproofing Boots

Don't. There are pros and cons about waterproofing. And I'm strictly on the con side. Waterproofed boots won't allow your feet to breathe freely. A healthy hike will cause your feet to perspire, wetting your socks and feet in non-breathable boots. And wet feet blister easily. Breathable boots, on the other hand, will allow perspiration to wick out while you hike. I'd rather my feet have a minimal amount of perspiration. If my socks do get wet and my feet begin to blister, I carry a supply of moleskin for such occasions. I allow my boots to dry naturally at night to reduce any foot odor.

Breaking In Boots

Before you wear new boots on the trail, be sure to break them in to be positive you're made the right decision. Wear them at home where the soles won't get soiled. Be sure to put on the socks you'll wear on the trail. This enables you to be doubly sure of their fit. Once you're sure they're right for you, then begin the breaking in process in earnest. Wear the boots on a few short hikes to allow them to conform to the subtleties of your feet. If you need professional orthotics, be sure to use them all during your fittings, and especially during your breaking-in period.

Despite my warning, there will be some who will still wait to buy their boots just before leaving on a week-long backpacking trip. They'll put on their new boots at the trailhead for the first time. I hope you aren't one of them. Nonetheless, I'm not one who would pass up a weeklong hike if there were no alternative but wearing a new pair of un-broken-in boots! So, enjoy. The hike will be worth it despite the blisters. However, do take along a supply of moleskin.

Trekking Poles

Hiking poles are relatively new to hiking. I first saw French hikers using their ski poles on glacial impacted trails in the Swiss Alps in the early 90s. Until recently I hiked with a simple Alpine hiking stick. But a few years ago (in my eighties) I bought hiking poles for stream crossings and rough trail. In the years since I've been using them, they've probably saved me from a few falls. So, I've become a strong advocate for us geezers to use hiking poles on even the easiest hikes. (See Chapter 8, *How Hiking Can Prevent Seniors from Falling.*) If you still have good balance, and haven't taken a fall for the past couple of years, you might get started hiking without them. However, you still may want to get poles for stream crossings and rougher terrain. And like me, you might even prevent a fall with hiking poles. The older I become, the fewer risks I'm willing to take. I'm kind of enjoying being alive and well enough to take daily hikes.

There's not a lot of difference among hiking pole brands. The ones I see most on the trail are like my Black Diamonds. Allow me to give you one tip on buying hiking poles. Choose the *mid-price* range pole from whichever brand you like. You don't need a lot of extra gadgets on the poles. Just that the poles be sturdy and feel good in your hands. Oh, and they should be adjustable. Get some advice from the sales clerk about how to adjust them.

How to Fit Your Hiking Pole Length

A good rule of thumb is to bend your arm at the elbow and hold your forearm level with the ground. Ask someone to see you bend your arm level to the ground. Doing it alone can be deceptive. Then adjust the length of the poles so that they fit comfortably in your hand when you hold them in that position. Don't worry about erring. You can re-adjust them whenever you like. That's why you're buying "adjustable" poles. After you use them a while, you may want to tweak them to a better length. When I found the correct length for me, it felt awkward at first. But after a while that pole length helped my posture. Their use at this length eliminated some butt pains I was beginning to develop.

Daypacks & Fanny Packs

You'll want a backpack or a fanny pack for carrying a few items on your hikes. It's your preference. If you are just becoming acquainted with hiking you really don't need either for your first hikes. You won't need a pack until you are taking hour-long hikes. Until then, the likeliest item you may want to carry is water. For short hikes, you can carry a plastic bottle of water in your hand. Of course, you might just want to take the plunge and buy a pack right at the beginning. As soon as you've decided that you're going to be a serious hiker, you've probably already made your choice. If you haven't, go to a good sporting goods store and discuss the matter with a knowledgeable sales clerk. My wife and I have Osprey daypacks. But it is just one of several good brands. Try some on. See which pack feels right for you.

Water

Water is the most important item you'll want to carry with you. How much water you need to drink depends on several things, such as how long you'll hike, how strenuous the trail, the weather and your age. A guideline for a sixty-year-old geezer in moderate weather, on a medium difficult trail, is about a half quart of water per hour of hiking. And to drink about a half pint of water before your hike as well as another half pint after the hike. The best practice for drinking for hiking is to take many small drinks rather than a few big ones. If you are just getting started, taking short beginner walks of a half hour or less, it's a good practice to have a water bottle in your car. Take a good drink just before your hike. Leave the bottle in your car and be sure to drink again after your hike. Taking both these drinks at your car relieves you of the necessity of carrying a water bottle on a short hike. I still do this. I leave my water bottle in the car for before and after drinks. For hikes of an hour or more, though, I carry water to drink along the trail. If in doubt, better to err by drinking more water, rather than less.

Ways To Carry Water

A. Canteens

The canteen is the old standard of foot soldier, Boy Scout, Campfire Girl and Intrepid Hiker! There is a great variety, at several price points, on the Internet. A nice thing about canteens is they usually have a carrying case and strap to hang over your shoulder for ease of access.

B. Plastic bottles of water

Store-bought bottles of water seem *de rigueur* for hikers out here. I see many hikers holding one of these water bottles in hand as they amble along a trail.

C. The 'Designer' Water Bottle

You may want to consider an environmentally friendly water bottle. They come in glass bottles, adequately covered by a thick rubber jacket to protect them from breakage, thus avoiding use of throwaway plastic bottles, which cause environmental problems.

D. Daypacks with Built-in Water Bladder

A backpack maker, Camelbak, some years ago developed a pack with a sewn-in water bladder. These packs have thin tubing running from the bladder to a spigot attached to the shoulder strap at chin level for convenience of drinking while hiking. Several companies have followed suit, making their own version of the Camelbak. I'm sure it's a convenience for drinking while hiking instead of stopping for rests along your route. I've never indulged, inasmuch as I like rest stops, and take many more than most hikers. An important reason I'm out in the woods is to spend some idle time soaking in the woodland energies.

Water Warnings

Do not drink water from streams or ponds unless you sterilize it. It's no longer like what it was in pioneering days.

First aid kit

It's good practice to bring along a first aid kit in your pack. There are myriad good options at sporting good stores.

Rainy Weather

There are arguments, very sound ones, against hiking in blue jeans and cotton shirts. When cotton gets wet from rain or body perspiration, it loses its capacity to keep you warm. In fact, these fabrics suck away your body's warmth, making you even colder. On the other hand, I like blue jeans and loose-fitting breathable cotton shirts for hikes of about an hour or so. They are comfortable. Should it rain, or I get wet in a creek, I believe I can suffer for the time it takes me to get back to my car and turn on the heater. Of course, the denim naysayers are right. Their choice of synthetic fabrics gives them a wide set of options, best told by knowledgeable clerks in sporting goods stores. If I'm going on a longer hike of a few hours or more, I wear good synthetic fabric clothing. In fact, on hot summer days, the synthetics are cooler than jeans.

Carry an Umbrella

My first editor of *Backpacker*, Laura Waterman, was an ardent proponent of the umbrella. Unless you are in gale force winds, it's a good, inexpensive rainy day option. For most easy hikes, the number one choice is one of those small folding umbrellas. It'll fit easily into your daypack and keep you dry should you be surprised by rain.

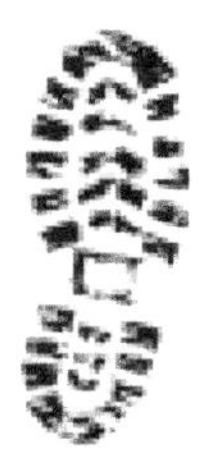

Chapter 6

Hiking Safely

Most likely as a geezer your *greatest* risk while hiking will be *yourself.* With age, you are prone to over-exertion, not realizing you really aren't as fit as you think you are. So be aware! Your next highest risk will be the same as what you have at home – medical issues. You will be further from medical assistance if an issue occurs on a hike.

Walking vs Hiking

The difference between 'walking' and 'hiking' is a good question about which to split hairs. I *walk* along a country road. But I *hike* the Divisadero Trail. I cover the same distance on the road as on the trail. So*, the difference* in my walking or hiking? My country road is a level surface with very little change in elevation. The Divisadero Trail, though, climbs 2,000 feet over rough rocky tread. How steep and rough does a path have to be to make a difference between a walk and a hike? After ninety, call it as you wish!

The question arose the other morning while I trudged along an easy trail. It occurred to me, of course, that hiking has a greater risk of tripping and falling. On the other hand, hiking builds those little muscles that enable me to catch myself when I do trip. It is much better than stair climbing, which provides as much, or even more, aerobic exercise than hiking. But stairs don't challenge those itty-bitty leg and feet muscles that go into action when I get a little off balance.

With that opening, let's begin by walking before you take up hiking. Then gradually advance to hiking on easy trails. Let your good judgment be your guide. Try not to do too much in too short a time. Nor doing too little.

Easy Does It

Don't just go right out onto a hike if you haven't hiked in years. And don't take a hike that you know challenges your physical ability. Put your ego on the shelf. Go hiking for enjoyment. Not to prove anything. I make this suggestion, knowing how difficult it is to keep my ego from taking charge of my hikes! For example, immediately following open-heart surgery, I had to gradually get back into hiking as a beginner. I had to start all over again. I was allowed to take only fifteen-minute walks along our country road. It took time, from walking daily along our country road, to gradually work my way up to short hikes on easy trails. Finally, I was able to hike moderately difficult trails without concern. It was all about being *realistic* about how much strain I should put on my heart.

Check with your doctor. Be sure your physical condition is up to the type of hike or walk you want to take. Find out, too, what the maximum heart rate is for someone your age, in your physical condition. I provide a lot of good information about this in other chapters of this book.

Let Someone Know Where You Will be Hiking

This is probably the most important, though least heeded, precaution for geezers. It is so easy to overlook this step. Especially when we feel real energetic. We tend to be optimistic and take our well-being for granted as we head out for a hike on a warm, sunny day. But, it takes just a short note about where you will go and when you expect to be back. I still do it today. My wife knows where I'll be hiking and when to expect my return. Be on the safe side. Have someone reliable know where you will be hiking. And when you'll be back. Also, what to do if you aren't back at that time. This is an especially important precaution for geezers.

Keep Trail Conversation to a Minimum

Of course we enjoy gabbing with friends when we get together. But chatting while hiking is a distraction that adds an unnecessary risk to your hike. It's better and more enjoyable to chat with a companion at rest stops where you can give each other full attention. I know, this goes against advice in most hiking handbooks, including my own, *Backpacker & Hikers' Handbook*. These handbooks usually suggest carrying on a conversation while hiking as a way of monitoring your heart rate. It's good advice. But more for younger hikers. After all, *we are geezers.* And we need to tweak a few of the rules for energetic youngsters to adjust for our age. When geezers carry on conversations while hiking it diverts our attention from the trail, which puts us at risk of taking a tumble. It's not easy to remember. I have a top-notch hiking friend who forgot. Madeline got caught up in trail conversation and suffered the consequences. In her younger days Madeline was a champion triathlete, and was still in top-notch shape as a geezer. But while concentrating on conversation she lost her footing and severely twisted an ankle. It meant enduring excruciating pain while her partner hiked out to get help. The risk of a twisted ankle, of course, is reduced appreciably when you're strolling along a road or sidewalk. Use your better judgment.

Water

It's another risk for geezers. Carry a good-size bottle of water on hikes of more than a half-hour. Drink your fill before setting out on the hike, as well as another good-size drink at the end. Develop such a drinking habit from the get-go. Geezers tend to dehydrate more than younger hikers. As we age our skin dries more quickly and our sense of thirst is slower. So we need to push ourselves to drink more often.

Why Our Bodies Dehydrate More as We Age

As we age our thirst factor does not kick in early enough for our drinking to rehydrate us. Thus, we need to drink more often than normal, especially when we hike.

According to sports medicine specialist, Dr. Emily Harold, we geezers dehydrate more for three reasons. Our body's flesh shrinks leaving less cellular capacity for water. We have a slower thirst response, which doesn't tell us we're thirsty until after the body already needs it. And our kidney function decreases with age, causing us to pass more water when we urinate than our body can afford to lose. Then, of course, we dehydrate more when we hike. Bottom line: we need to drink a good bit more water than younger people, especially while hiking. And we ought to sip frequently as we hike rather than drink large amounts less often.

Use Two Hiking Poles

I first saw hikers using ski poles years ago while hiking in the Swiss Alps. Today, hiking poles are commonplace everywhere. I'd bet half of the geezers I see on the trails out here are using them. A few summers ago while I was still wed to my Swiss alpenstock, I was hiking a trail where we had to make several stream crossings on stepping-stones. With my usual self-confidence I stepped from the bank of the stream out onto a stepping-stone for our first stream crossing. The stone rocked and I rocked with it, landing on my butt in the stream. Luckily, I only got wet, had a skinned elbow and great embarrassment. A skilled hiker like me! Need help getting up out of the water onto my feet! No way! Okay! Just *a little* help.

My wife insisted that while she wouldn't mind my dying while doing what I love most, she'd hate to see me wheelchair-bound, unable to get back out onto a trail any more. So of course I was lucky enough to learn my lesson. I bought my first pair of hiking poles. At first, I used them just for stream crossings; though shortly I found them useful for other tricky, trail maneuvers. It didn't take much longer to find them useful on all my hikes. Today I wouldn't hike without them. Even on the easiest trails. I've confessed this here so that I can't be accused of any "do as I say, not as I do" advice. In fact, I simply could not have survived my recent sciatic episodes without my hiking poles.

Hike With a Friend

It's all right to walk alone when you have sufficient trail experience. It is always best, though, to hike with a partner. You will see many hikers going alone, even running on more popular trails, these days. Okay, if you are that advanced, you probably aren't reading this book. While most of us would like a trail companion, it's not easy to come by one. If you do find a good trail friend, still be prepared to hike by yourself when your companion can't or 'just isn't up for a hike.' For that will be the quickest way to fail in your resolve to become a regular hiker. Nonetheless, hiking with a partner is still safer than going alone.

If you can't find a hiking companion, then go for a walk. Don't hike. It's much safer. Be patient. Especially with yourself. Why not enjoy your last years of life? If you don't stay at it, you'll probably miss the healthiest and easiest exercise possible. And suffer several ailments of old age as a result. And here is encouraging advice: According to the American Heart Association, walking is the one exercise with the greatest number of people sticking to it.

Hike Safe Trails

Pick easy, popular trails on which there are sure to be other hikers. This practice assures you that if you have an emergency, someone will come along who can go for help or comfort you while someone else does. I gave up hiking solo on remote trails that may lack help should I need it. I loved my solo excursions over many hiking years. And I would still love them if it weren't for the wisdom I've accrued as I've aged.

Know When to Turn Back

Get over it! You need ~~to~~ prove nothing. It's not wussy to say, "Guys, it's been fun. But it's time for me to turn back." Be honest with yourself, your age and weather conditions, and you will enjoy hiking more than you ever imagined. One day recently as I was coming down the South Boundary Trail, I heard a guy tell his hiking friend just that. He'd only hiked in maybe half a mile. He was seated breathlessly on a rock beside the trail. His face was flushed, shirt wet with perspiration. He looked to be in his late thirties or early forties. He was honest enough with himself and his friend to avoid risking a heart attack. I've turned back early on many, many occasions over the years. Recently three of us turned back early because of weather conditions. No big deal! We were out to enjoy ourselves. And we wanted to continue enjoying ourselves for as many years as possible. We have nothing to prove — except to prove to ourselves that we can keep on hiking and enjoying it.

Carry Basic Necessities In Your Pack

When you have built your body sufficiently for longer hikes, you'll want to carry a daypack with at least the following items.

1. Water
2. Rain gear
3. First aid kit
4. Your medications
5. High-carb snacks

This minimal list presumes that you are hiking no more than two or three hours. When you become more serious, and head out for more than a few hours, you ought to carry "The Ten Essentials" that outfitters recommend. Here are REI's recommendations: (https://www.rei.com/content/dam/documents/pdf/Gear Checklists/PrinterFriendly/REI_Expert_Advice_Day_Hiking_Checklist.pdf) Of course, when you are hiking at this level of experience, you will definitely want more essentials in your pack. You'll know when you have this much experience. And have a good idea of all that you need to carry.

Chapter 7

How Fit Are You?

While you may not be in the greatest physical condition, you are probably still fit enough to take a fifteen-minute walk on an easy path every day. It might save you from an early death from a sedentary life-style, which is being found to be a higher risk for geezers than a heart attack or stroke. I'm, of course, suggesting you take up hiking, which is just a notch above walking, as an enjoyable life-saving exercise.

~~~~~~

Warning: being out of shape is a greater risk of death than heart attack, stroke, diabetes and falling.
(See: https://www.cnn.com/2018/10/19/health/study-not-exercising-worse-than-smoking/index.html)

~~~~~~

Being In Shape Has Some Very Practical Benefits.

One benefit is how it keeps you from serious injuries. My hiking partner Erik goes a step farther. Erik Steinberg was an Olympic ski coach and puts it this way: "Physical fitness *equals* injury prevention." He claims to have proved it in real time. In coaching the first American US Olympic alpine ski champions, Erik instructed them in how to race at 100 mph speeds while avoiding injuries that would put them out of the competition as well as possibility incapacitating them for life.

So, think simply, 'easy does it.' Easy enough to *want to do it.*

How Fit Are You?

This would be a good place to stop and take inventory of your physical condition. What shape are you *really* in? Not what shape do you *think* you are in! You shouldn't be thinking about how far or how fast you *can* hike. It ought to be about getting an honest fix on the shape you are in right now. Even a couple of years of inactivity as you age can make a significant difference in your physical fitness.

Let's face it. It isn't easy to appraise our own physical condition. It's natural for us to think we can still do what we did just two to three years ago. But can we? It really is wisest to err on the safer side.

How About a Spa or Class?

There are many classes and physical fitness programs, as well as gyms and spas where professionals can give you a good fitness once-over. I've tried a few and they were good. Some even offer walking groups. Years ago when my office was in the middle of Manhattan, I took a physical fitness program at noon daily. The class was held daily and we could come as often or infrequently as we liked. To get into the class, we had to pass a physical examination right there at the club given by the in-house physician assistant. Classes like these can be beneficial. The "Silver Sneakers" program that many insurance companies offer senior clients are also worthwhile. Nonetheless, while these programs often produce good results, I'm still urging you to take up hiking. And all you really need is a pair of sneakers. And of course, your doctor's okay. Hiking is such an enjoyable option that it will out-last these other programs. Studies show that walking, especially hiking, is the best and easiest way to better health. Furthermore, it is proven that most people who begin a walking or hiking program are most likely to stay with it over the long haul.

Physical Fitness Tests

It isn't necessary for you to have an overall physical fitness assessment of yourself for you to take up hiking. But it will help you avoid injuries. There are many good tests to see how fit you are before beginning a hiking regimen. Here's a good one to begin with that may have the most beneficial effect for your walking. It builds strength in your legs.

Chair Rise Exercise

The U.S. Center for Disease Control (CDC) suggests a Chair Rise Exercise to both test the strength of the muscles in your thighs and buttocks and to build strength. (See https://www.cdc.gov/steadi/pdf/Chair_Rise_Exercise-print.pdf.)

You do this test simply by standing up from a sitting position. And sitting back down. Everyone can pass this test if they are able to stand up from sitting on a standard height table chair. There are degrees of difficulty depending upon where you place your hands as you lift yourself up from the chair.

1. Sit toward the front of the chair, your knees bent and feet flat on the floor. Keep your feet shoulder-width apart.
2. Rest your hands on the seat slightly to each side of you. Keep your back and neck straight, and chest slightly forward.
3. Breathe in slowly. Lean forward and feel your weight on the front of your feet.
4. Breathe out slowly. Then slowly stand up, using your hands as little as possible.
5. Pause while you are still standing. Take a full, deep breath, in and back out.
6. Breathe in as you slowly sit back down. Do not allow yourself to collapse back into the chair. Control yourself as much as you can while lowering yourself slowly back down into the chair.

The CDC has illustrations and exercise recommendations for how to build muscle strength from this exercise.

A Simple Overall Fitness Self-Test

I've used this simple self-testing program from time to time. It is a set of six simple exercise tests that you can do at home for quick results. They were developed years ago for the President's Physical Fitness Council, but don't let the simplicity fool you. They were developed for younger adults. And you will not likely pass many of them. However, they will give you a picture of where you need to focus corrective attention. And they'll help motivate you to get started on the easiest and most helpful fitness program.

I have again and again failed to pass a couple of them, even though I've been doing the suggested remedial exercises for years. So, should you take these tests, don't be surprised at the results. As I said, I still have not passed a couple of them, though I won't tell you which. One good thing about these tests is that there is a very easy set of exercises that take less than fifteen minutes a day to correct your performance. They are spelled out in Hans Kraus' classic book on back aches, *Backache, Stress, and Tension: Understanding Why You Have Back Pain and Simple Exercises to Prevent and Treat It.* Dr. Kraus explains how, with illustrations, and why you ought to do these exercises, especially to treat and prevent backaches. Dr. Hans Kraus, the author of the book, and Sonja Weber of New York Presbyterian Hospital developed the tests.

Exercise One

The first exercise is to do one simple sit-up. Lay flat on your back on the floor, knees bent and feet flat. Have someone hold your feet. Or place them beneath a heavy enough object to hold them while doing the exercise. Clasp your hands behind your head and gently, slowly sit up. Do not jerk yourself up. It may cause unnecessary strain.

Exercise Two

This exercise is a variation of the first. This time perform the same sit-up with your legs extended with knees not bent. Again, with your hands clasped behind your head, roll up gently and slowly into the sit-up. This exercise with straight legs lessens the hip flexors and puts more emphasis on the abdominal muscles.

Exercise Three

For the third exercise, lie flat on your back, legs straight. Now raise your feet about eight inches off the ground. Hold the position for 10 seconds. Inability to keep your feet raised or if you have to significantly arch your back to keep your feet elevated is to fail the test.

Exercise Four

Lie on your stomach with a pillow beneath your pelvis; clasp your hands behind your head. Have someone hold your feet and pelvis down. Now raise your head, chest and shoulders up off the floor. Hold the position for 10 seconds. The exercise tests your upper back muscles.

Exercise Five

This exercise starts in the same position as Exercise Four. This time have someone hold your upper back and shoulders to keep your chest on the floor. Keep your feet together while you lift your legs off the floor. Hold them up for 10 seconds. The exercise tests your lower back muscles.

Exercise Six

Standing, feet together and arms by your side. With your knees straight, bend slowly forward to touch the floor. Remain in that position for three seconds. It's an exercise to test your overall flexibility, especially your back muscles.

How to Avoid or Treat a Backache

Probably the most common issue that we geezers suffer is backaches. And the most common cure is surgery. I'm not a doctor, so what I have to say may not apply to your condition. However, it has been suggested by two of my physician friends, one of whom, Dr. Hans Kraus of the Kraus-Weber Tests, was the orthopedic surgeon who was the only doctor who managed to help President John F. Kennedy with his back pains. Both doctors suggested I "avoid the knife" for relieving the pain of my herniated discs. MRI's showed that I have two herniated discs.

The first chapter of Dr. Kraus' book, *The Cause, Prevention and Treatment of BACKACHE, Stress and Tension,* gives a really easy set of exercises to correct the failure to pass each of the tests. He suggests a pattern of continued exercises to stay in shape. *And most important, he suggests an additional set of exercises to correct backaches, which are geezers' most common physical complaint.*

If You Decide On Surgery

Your surgeon will probably separate the muscles and nerves that are causing your back to ache, but unless you take corrective action, these muscles and nerves frequently migrate back to the same troublesome configuration that caused your back to ache in the first place. Dr. Kraus' exercises will help you to stave off this return. *Approach your hiking not for how much you can do, but as a prescription for a longer, healthier, more enjoyable life.*

Chapter 8

How Hiking Can Prevent Seniors from Falling, A Review

As I trudged up the Divisadero Trail one day recently the thought arose, that 'yes, hiking does a lot more than I realized to keep me from falling!' It's why I'm touting hiking as even better than walking for keeping my balance.

So, When Does Walking Become Hiking?

There is a noticeable difference between my 'walking' and my 'hiking.' I *walk* a mile along our country road, which is good exercise. But I *hike* a mile up the Divisadero Trail. It's the same distance, but with an important difference. Our road has a smooth surface with gentle slopes. The Divisadero Trail though, has an uneven, rocky tread and some stretches of steep climbing. That difference is important for preventing falls. Hiking the trail exercises a variety of minuscule leg, ankle and feet muscles that help my balance and are not exercised as much in walking the road. Hiking also utilizes subtle ways in which my body's balancing mechanisms are engaged when scrambling over roots and rocks.

Hiking is also better for my balance than climbing stairs. It's true that stair climbing provides as much, or even better, aerobic exercise than hiking. But climbing stairs doesn't exercise those intricate muscles used in scrambling over roots and rocks, the muscles that go into action when my balance tilts a little off kilter.

Why Falling Is So Lethal for Seniors

This might be a good place to talk about why we geezers are more and more prone to falling, the older we become. The risk is two-edged. The older we are the more often we fall. And falls become more serious with age! So, let me bring up the numbers before I get into how to dodge the risks.

The Serious Odds of Falling

1. One out of four geezers over 65 will take a fall this year. You may fall at home, while shopping, socializing, walking or even while hiking. If you are lucky enough not to take a fall this year, you still aren't out of the woods.
2. Each year after geezers reach 65, they are going to face the same odds – one of every four is going to take a tumble. And those odds are the same, year after year, for the rest of our lives. No let up!
3. And the risk of falling is even greater for women than men.
4. Half the geezers who fall and aren't injured, nonetheless, cannot get up without assistance.
5. Taking a fall is the reason most geezers will be admitted to a hospital for a serious injury.
6. But still, the leading cause of geezers dying from an injury is falling.
7. The number of geezers who fracture their hip from a fall also increases each year as we grow older.
8. One out of ten of us who live past 85 will fracture a hip from a fall. And those numbers increase with each year we get older.
9. *Worse still*: one in four geezers who fracture a hip will die within six months of that injury!
10. And falls, with or without injury, can radically change the quality of our life. Even the loss of our independent living.

How Hiking Helped Me Beat the Odds

While nine of ten geezers my age have lost their independent living, I'm fortunate to be beating the odds and still hiking daily. And I believe it is mostly because for some time I have been taking a hike every day.

Fear's Double-Edged Sword

A growing number of geezers, when they find out about these risks, fear falling so much that they limit their physical activity to avoid them. But, lack of activity, in turn, results in further physical decline. And this is almost always accompanied by depression, social isolation, and a feeling of helplessness. If you follow my easy-does-it approach to hiking, you should not only avoid this grim scenario, but also help prevent your falling and enable you to enjoy better health as well.

After the Hard Facts, Let's Get Back to Hiking.

The hardest part of taking a hike is lacing up your boots and heading out the door. I mean it. It's difficult to get started. When I had open-heart surgery, the doctors forced me to walk as soon as I awoke from the ether. And I only wanted to go back to sleep! They put me on my feet as soon as I came out of the anesthetic and had me walking down the hall, propped up by nurse on each side of me. I didn't walk far. It was very unpleasant! But I *was* walking. So, I do know how difficult getting started on a walk can be. When they sent me home three days later, they told me to walk fifteen minutes every day. I know! That's very easy walking. But not so easy just four days after this surgery. They'd sawed open my chest. Taken out my heart. Set it on an autopilot machine. Then cut big chunks of arteries from my legs. Sewed them onto gaps in my heart's arteries where they'd cut out the clogging sections. Of course, they then stitched me back together again. They then, just four days later, wanted *me* to get up out of bed on my own and *go for a walk*? Really! I've got a persuasive wife, though. So I walked, and watched every minute of those first fifteen click by. In time though, I didn't mind. And I increased my walking to twenty minutes a day. Then walking twenty-five. And eventually, thirty minutes every day. For, as Sir Isaac Newton said, "Things *in motion* tend to stay *in motion*." But its opposite, as well, "Things *at rest* tend to stay *at rest*."

Five Ways to Make Hiking Keep You Safer from Falling

Most importantly, frequent hiking helps you keep your balance and avoid a fall.

1. *Make a habit first of walking daily.*

Regardless of your physical condition, begin your program by taking a short, fifteen-minute walk *every day*. Do this, even if you are already an occasional hiker. This is important. It's easy. So do it.

There's nothing wrong with continuing to take longer, occasional hikes as well. But I'm repeating! You can count an occasional hike as your daily walk. But days you aren't hiking, then take that fifteen-minute walk. Develop it into a firm *daily* routine. Make it so easy to take that walk that it doesn't go the way of a New Year's resolution. Just walk *only fifteen* minutes a day. Even if you are still working at a regular job, you can find fifteen minutes some place in your day to walk for fifteen minutes. Lunchtime, after work, even before work. No matter how many hours of work you do in a day. No matter where you are. Even in a hotel away on business. You can still take a walk. Even in street clothes and street shoes. You can still take a daily walk. This is a great habit to develop *before* you retire. You will be in great shape for hiking daily when you do retire. After a while, very gradually, increase the amount of time you walk. Wait until you feel the time is right, before substituting a short hike on an easy trail, for your daily walk. Be patient with yourself. We're talking now about your life! Keep on taking your short walks until it becomes a habit to take them. Get real used to walking. And when it is firmly established as a habit, only then substitute hiking for the walking. Try to find the joy of the outdoors in your daily walking. It is a great soothing respite from a hectic schedule.

One Further Dictum:

Don't give yourself the excuse not to take your daily walk because "You've been on your feet all day." You must be intentional to form a habit. So no matter how much you've been on your feet, nor how far you've had to walk during the day, you must specifically *intend* to take your daily walk. Set aside all other thoughts about your day's activity and tell yourself, "I am now going to take my daily walk," as you start walking, even if it is no more than five minutes. It has to be intentional to form the habit. It will help you turn your *intention* into an *actual* "daily walk." It might even help if you remind yourself of what it takes to pave the road to Hell.

2. Go more slowly than you think you need to.

Walking is absolutely the best exercise for a longer, healthier life. It's the easiest exercise you can do because it is so natural. You walk because you have two legs. The beauty of walking and hiking is that you get as much aerobics as you need without trying. This makes 'sauntering' enjoyable, especially for us geezers. For we need not struggle trying to do more than is comfortable. For reasons such as this, it is the easiest habit to sustain once you develop it. Don't take my word for it. These are American Heart Association findings.

Let your daily hike become a prime fitness purpose of your life. Making it a purpose is powerful. Studies at Mount Sinai St. Luke's Medical Center show that people, regardless of age, who have a purpose in their lives have a 77-percent chance of avoiding dying *from all causes*. With daily hiking as a high purpose in your life you will also benefit in two distinct ways. Honestly. You'll have better health. And you'll live longer.

3. *Hike with trekking poles.*

When you shift from walking to hiking, be sure to use a pair of ski-pole-type hiking poles. They improve balance and even give your arms a boost, loosening them and gradually strengthen them as well. You may even want to begin using hiking poles while walking, before you begin hiking.

4. *While hiking, and even walking, do less talking.*

Give your attention fully to where you are stepping. Any missed step, can cause a fall. It is best to save conversation for your rest stops. You do not want a single miss-step. Not even on a road. And certainly not on a rocky trail.

5. *Easy does it.*

Don't go for the gold. Easy does it. Don't hike to prove how fast or how far you can go. Nor to get ahead of someone. Hike for the joy of being out in the open air. And if you *don't* feel joyful, *pretend* you do. For there is an old maxim that says, "Change an action to change a mood."

Instead of trying to hike faster and farther, simply try to make hiking a daily habit. Consistency counts far more than hiking achievements. It's a lot easier to remember to do something every day, than it is to remember it two or three times a week. And of course, there are bound to be days when something more important does come up. Oftentimes though, you can shift your hike to a different time of day. Otherwise, you may have to just miss a day's hike. From time to time, I have a doctor's appointment in Albuquerque. It is a 2-1/2 hour drive each way from my home in Taos. When I add in the time it takes with the doctor I've been gone the better part of the day. So hiking is usually not practical on those days, except in mid-summer when days are longer. Nonetheless, hiking daily is easier than trying to remember whether you decided to hike on say, Tuesdays and Fridays or Mondays and Thursdays.

Risks of Falling While Hiking in the Rain

While you probably won't start out on a hike in the rain, there will be times when you get caught in a downpour before you finish. And of course, risks of falling are greater during the rain. So take the following precautions

1. Don't worry about getting wet.

Your only concern during a rainstorm ought to be caution about where and how you take the next step along the trail. Not whether you get wet. I wear synthetic fiber clothing whenever possible. And I carry nothing in my pockets that matters if it gets wet. It's usually just my driver's license and my medical insurance card, both of which are plastic coated. Oh, and my car keys. So, I don't need to worry about getting drenched when I get caught in the rain. I can therefore focus full attention on where I am stepping so that I won't take a tumble.

2. Don't rush.

There is always a temptation when the first raindrops fall to hurry to get to shelter as soon as possible. This can be particularly dangerous. The trail you've been safely hiking will present new risks. Rocks and pebbles that gave you good footing when the sun was out, become treacherously slippery when wet and muddy. I'm emphasizing this, for after years and years of hiking, I still want to rush back to the car when I'm caught in the rain. I know though, that this impulse must be held in check to be sure I take extra caution about where and how I take my next step.

3. Step more carefully

A downhill slope can be your most trying and risky section and sloping trail tread begs for special caution in the rain. It is an invitation to a slippery surprise. And the older you get the worse a fall.

Try not to walk sideways down a slippery slope, unless of course, you can get obvious footholds. The best way is to find rock outcroppings for footholds to work your way down. Tread carefully for they, too, can be slippery. If you must step in mud or gravel then do it flatfooted with your toes pointed downhill. It will give you better foot-gripping power.

Chapter 9

Find Your Comfortable Hiking Pace

As we age, we geezers find it increasingly difficult to keep up with other hikers. But, it is critical that you find out how to deal with this. It could save your life. We all have a safe hiking comfort zone. This is a good time to find out yours. And, once you find it, stick to it no matter who you are hiking with. There's nothing wussy about it. John Muir, the mountain man founder of the Sierra Club, said he even hated the word 'hike.'. . . we "ought to saunter in the mountains. Not 'hike!' " So, if sauntering was good enough for that old hiker, shouldn't it be good enough for us old geezers, too?

So How to Adjust Your Hiking Pace When You Least Want to

We all walk naturally within our personal comfort zone. It is a safe pace at which to hike. Especially hiking longer distances. There's an easy way to find your own comfort zone. Whether you can stick to it while hiking with others, though, will take an attitude adjustment. And that isn't so easy. I have found that the more I hike at my comfortable pace, the less likely I'm bothered keeping up with faster hikers. Even with my wife and young friends. You too, will probably feel more relaxed lagging behind faster hikers once you've mastered sauntering in your personal comfort zone.

Four Suggestions

1. How to find your hiking comfort zone.

Start by taking a hike by yourself. Finding your safe hiking comfort zone is critical as you age. It's not easy for us to find it. And generally it's way too difficult to "be ourself" while hiking with others. The younger you are, the more difficult it will be for you to even want to know your comfort pace. It flies in the face of our culture's "can-do" attitude. But, consider the consequences of taking your immortality for granted.

2. Find a less-traveled road.

Measure off a mile of the road with your car's odometer and mark both ends of it. Flag a tree at each end, for instance.Comfortably walk the distance between the two points. Time how long it takes. Walk the same distance again on another day, to be sure of your measurement. Let that be your base-line hiking pace on level ground. For much of my hiking life this was somewhat more than three miles per hour. As I entered my geezer years, this slipped to 2-1/2 miles per hour, or 24 minutes per mile. Recently though, it dropped even more. I'm often hiking at about two miles an hour, or 30 minutes per mile. That's okay. It's what is comfortable for me. There is no "right" pace for everyone. We're all a bit different. The most important thing is whether the pace is enjoyable for you. For if you insist on pushing it higher, it will become a drag on whether you want to get out to hike. And if you push it too high, for any sustained period, it might badly affect your well-being.

3. Add time to your pace for climbing/elevation gains

Add time to your comfortable pace for each thousand feet of elevation you need to climb. The Appalachian Mountain Club's *White Mountain Guide* calculates it takes the average hiker about an additional half hour per thousand feet of elevation gain. That's a comfortable amount of time for the "average hiker." Back in my backpacking days it was a sufficient calculation. But you are probably not the average hiker, and if you are getting up in age you need more time to climb a thousand feet. Today, because of my age, I allow an additional hour to climb a thousand feet. That means, to hike a mile while climbing a thousand feet, I need to add an hour for the climb to the half hour to hike a mile. A total of 1-1/2 hours to hike a mile up a thousand feet.

Become Intensely Aware of Your Hiking Pace While Hiking with Others

Be the last hiker in the group. Accept it if you lag behind at your slower pace. You'll enjoy yourself more. If you are with friends, they'll gladly stop from time to time to wait for you

Allow Other Hikers to Pass You on the Trail

Remind yourself that you are out to enjoy your hike. There is no one you need to impress. I tell you this as though it were easy. And it *is easy* for me to write about it. But, at first, it was very difficult to allow myself to hike at a slower pace when hiking with others. And it took awhile to get used to it. After all, because I'd been Editor of *Backpacker* magazine, other hikers expected me to be an uber-hiker. And back in the day I felt I had to try living up to their expectations.

I got over it. I ate a little humble-pie. I now have my comfortable sauntering pace, no matter with whom I'm hiking. Give it a try. See what happens. Practice has enabled me to thoroughly enjoy hiking regardless of the pace of others. And it doesn't matter much what others may think of my pace. In fact, you will find that, in time, people will actually admire you for your ability to throttle down.

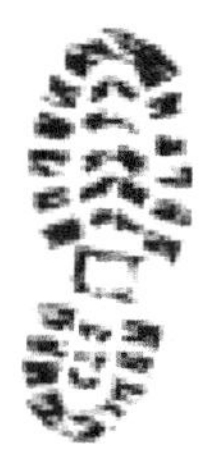

Chapter 10

Ten Health Benefits of Hiking

Health professionals give good reasons why hiking may be the best physical exercise for the health of your body and mind. There are even neuroscientists who claim walking is the best thing you can do to increase your brainpower.

1. *Hiking Reduces Your Risk of a Heart Attack.*

Heart disease is the number one cause of death. And the average age at the first heart attack is just over sixty-five for men and seventy-two for women. The American Heart Associations says walking [of which hiking is just a bit more strenuous] is the best way to stay away from the emergency room with a heart attack. They are basing their view on many studies. (See: http://www.heart.org/HEARTORG/HealthyLiving/PhysicalActivity/Walking/Walk-Don't-Run-Your-Way-to-a-Healthy-Heart_UCM_452926_Artle.jsp - .Wxm1h6knbBI)

2. *Hiking Substantially Reduces the Risk of Your Having a Stroke.*

Stroke is a serious concern for good reason. After a major stroke, survivors may become permanently disabled. Prevention is the best medicine for stroke. (See: https://www.health.harvard.edu/heart-health/walk-more-to-slash-your-stroke-risk.) One of life's most mundane activities — taking a walk — can significantly reduce your risk of stroke. Furthermore, the more hours a week you walk, even at a relaxed pace, the greater the odds you *will not* have a stroke. Several studies indicate that hiking prevents not just strokes, but many other maladies of our senior years. (See: https://www.webmd.com/fitness-exercise/features/hiking-body-mind)

3. Hiking Reduces Your Risk of Dying from Colon Cancer

Recent studies showed that hiking very likely reduced the number of colon cancer deaths among seniors. Researchers who studied levels of physical activity among 150,000 people with colon cancer showed those more physically active had a far lower number of colon cancer cases. As well, of course, far fewer deaths from colon cancer.

Dr. Kathleen Wolin at Washington University School of Medicine, who conducted this study, said that the greatest benefits showed among those who had exercised for the largest portion of their lives. But even among late starters the numbers were close as well. She said, "You get an enormous 'bang for the buck,' if you go for even a 30-minute walk every day." (See: https://www.telegraph.co.uk/news/health/news/8233508/ Walking-for-30-minutes-a-day-lowers-colon-cancer-risk.html)

4. Hiking Might Very Well Prevent Diabetes

Hiking uses up more energy, which reduces your blood sugar levels naturally. So it ought not to be a surprise that studies show that hiking can help prevent diabetes. Moreover, if you already have diabetes, hiking can help you manage it.

I have been a Type-2 diabetic for half of my life. And I've experienced dangerously "low" blood sugar levels on hikes more often than I like to admit. It is proof to me that I've been, unwittingly, using hiking to maintain reduced blood sugar levels. In fact, now is a good time to warn you about *low blood sugar levels*. Be sure to carry some high carb snacks, like a handful of Lifesavers, with you on every hike. Learn to recognize the symptoms of low blood sugar, like lightheadedness and lack of energy. *Be sure you still have time to quickly boost your blood sugar level should you feel faint, light-headed and weakened energy level. It can be fatal to wait too long to give your blood a sugar boost!*

5. Hiking Improves Balance, Preventing Falls

Falls are the biggest cause of fatality from injury in geezers over 65. And Lord knows, the older we become, the more prone we are to taking a tumble. I believe it is not just that we lose our balance as we age. It's that we don't seem able to avoid falling when we do lose balance. I've struggled with my balance for years. And I can readily see that I am losing it much more often as I get older. However, hiking has strengthened those tiny, subtle muscles in my ankles, legs and hips. It enables me to catch myself from falling when I do get slightly off balance. Studies show that, as we age and continue hiking we are more able to prevent ourselves from falling.

6. Hiking Is a Good Prescription for Mental Composure

I've found it difficult to hike with an unpleasant mood, for my mood seems to change in less than a hundred paces along a trail. Doctors in Japan are now writing prescriptions for patients to get out on a trail to 'forest bathe' as an anti-dote for emotional illness. Forest bathing isn't the same as hiking. It is just being out in a forest among the trees. There is a large forested area in Tokyo, Japan with trails for forest bathing. Its trailheads have signs that warn visitors to walk, not run, which really means the same as "hike, don't run," the numbers were close.

The Japanese did technical studies that say that just getting out into the woods we absorb a microbiotic antidote, called *phytonicide,* from the trees. It sounds to me that we get *aroma therapy* in the woods with a scientific name. There is a good book which is well worth reading just for motivation to get you outdoors if nothing else: *Forest Bathing: How Trees Can Help You Find Health and Happiness*. (See Chapter 2 for further details.)

I honestly believe that the main reason for my continued physical well-being on into my nineties, despite my many health issues, is my regular hiking. Hiking certainly has added to my continued upbeat attitude toward life.

7. Hiking May Make Us Brainier

According to a neuroscientist, Shane O'Mara, the human species was designed to be in motion. O'Mara has what he calls a 'motor-centric' idea of the brain. In other words, he thinks our brain was designed to get us into movement. And keep us there. Therefore, if we stop moving about, it stops us functioning properly. (See: https://www.theguardian.com/lifeandstyle/2019/jul/28/its-a-superpower-how-walking-makes-us-healthier-happier-and-brainier)

8. Hiking Is the Easiest Physical Exercise to Sustain

Study after study show that once we start a hiking program, we are likely to stick with it. The benefits are considerable no matter whether you are returning to the trail after years that career demands kept you away from the trails, or whether you are just now about to take your first hike. And this may prompt you to get your boots on. You can hike just about anywhere, even in congested cities, if only on a sidewalk.

9. You Don't Have to be in Shape to Hike

You can begin a hiking regimen no matter what your physical condition. Even if you are overweight or in poor health. You can begin slowly.-It can really improve your physical condition. Put all your excuses aside. You can always just take at least a 'walk around the block.' I didn't even let hospitalization be an excuse not to hike! So I 'hiked' the corridors of the hospital, carrying along the tubes they had plugged into me. The medics thought that getting out of bed and walking about gave me a speedier recovery.

10. Hiking Doesn't Require Special Training, Facilities or Equipment

Unlike other types of physical exercise, such as golf, tennis or swimming, you do not need any special equipment or facility to take a hike. Since you need no equipment, you are always prepared to take at least a walk around the block. The only equipment you need is a comfortable pair of shoes you could actually go out your door, dressed as you are, and take your first hike right now, even if it is just around the block.

Here is the American Heart Association on walking. And of course, hiking is just a small step more than walking. *"All you have to do is lace up a good pair of sneakers — and walk. It's that easy. It's also safe, the least expensive and has the lowest dropout rate of any type of exercise. "It's not a skill-dependent form of activity. It's the most accessible form of physical activity. You can do it almost anywhere." Before you know it, brisk walking can become a part of your daily routine. And you'll reap plenty of benefits."*

Chapter 11

Hiking With Diabetes

I've found that, like me, many of my geezer friends are diabetics. We've each had our share of issues that we had not anticipated nor taken appropriate precautions against. I have been a diabetic for over half my life and have had my episodes of high blood sugars. As well as my low blood sugar levels. So, right from the start, let me emphasize the seriousness of hiking with diabetes. I first want to give you the basics. And then I'll tell you a couple of stories about hikers who, but for coincidences, would have died due to their ignoring some basics about hiking with this disease. The first and most obvious consideration is to be sure to carry a sufficient supply of all your medications. Also take plenty of extra high-energy food items. Take more than what you expect to need. I like dried apricots or pineapple, for example. You may prefer high-energy bars. Whatever your choice, be sure It has extra carbohydrates. It's for emergencies. Not for ordinary consumption. If you are on insulin, be particularly attentive. Take along your insulin and syringes. But be careful not to inject too much. If I eat a high-carb lunch and I won't need any extra energy to hike, I can take a little less insulin than usual in my shot.

While you'll probably be especially cautious planning your backpacking jaunts, it is easy to become reckless on day hikes. Don't think for a minute you're out of the woods with what you already know about diabetes. Some of us also thought we did. And yet we ran into unforeseen miscalculations!

Be sure to take along your prescribed pills or insulin (both types), your glucose-monitoring meter, plenty of extra test strips and syringes. Take extra supplies of all your meds and supplies.

As a rule of thumb, in addition to my usual needs at home, I take three extra syringes for each day I'll be out on a trail, as well as extra vials of insulin. Imagine, for example, accidentally breaking or losing a vial of insulin, with another couple of days needed to finish a hike. Take my advice seriously. It is essential for your safety. And it may well save your life.

Watch Your Blood Sugar Levels

Your blood sugar levels will change radically while hiking. Hiking burns a good deal more energy than you may realize, but not as much as you may imagine!

Danger of Low Blood Sugar

At an early stage of my diabetes, I was naturally more concerned about high blood sugar levels. And I failed to consider how much energy I burn while hiking. Hence, one day I found out. I was climbing up a mountain ridge deep in the Wheeler Peak Wilderness Area. I began to feel sluggish. 'Okay,' I thought, 'I'm tired from the climb.' So, not wanting to be a wuss, I pushed on. Eventually, I felt so weak-kneed I didn't see how I could continue the climb. I was resting more often than hiking. Could my blood sugar be running low? I had taken my usual insulin shot with lunch earlier in the day. Had I known how much more energy it takes for strenuous climbing, I probably would not have taken my lunch-time insulin. I finally realized that my morning's hike had driven my blood sugar level dangerously low. Uh, oh! I needed carbohydrates. But, fast! It was crucial to get my blood sugar up! There was nothing more to eat in my pack. I suddenly realized how dangerous my condition had become. How long would it take me to hike back out! Yet, how perilously little energy I had left! And no way to replenish it! I panicked! I *should* have known better, of course! Thoughts flashed through mind — 'Got to get something sweet.' 'Gotta get back out!' ' 'Gotta go, FAST!' I was getting weaker by the minute. I stumbled dumbly along the trail. I must have looked drunk. I didn't dare sit down for fear I'd not be able to get back up. I hoped I'd meet another hiker. Beg for something to eat. But I didn't see a soul. It took every bit of my resolve to push myself on and on and on. Finally back out to my car. Luckily I found a banana I'd *miraculously* left in the car. It was sufficient to raise my blood sugar enough to drive into the nearest town where I chugged a giant Coca Cola and gobbled an apricot empanada, a deliciously sweet Hispanic pastry stuffed with apricot preserves.

Being the founder of *Backpacker* magazine and author of books on hiking, I ought to have known better! My lesson, of course, was to never again hike without extra high-energy snacks in my pack. Especially on day hikes, on which I always seem to underestimate the difficulty.

Risk of High Blood Sugar

Having now confessed my *low* blood sugar episode, here's another. A *high* blood sugar story. It too, is about someone who ought to have known better. Our need to be concerned about too much sugar in our blood ought to be obvious. Especially to a physician. Right? My friend, Alison, a retired heart surgeon, told me this story. He had a friend who almost croaked on a backpacking trip in Wyoming's Wind River Mountains. They'd backpacked into a lovely spot. They set up camp and prepared dinner. And while waiting for its preparation, they each had a drink. It had been a joyous day. Until Alison's friend complained of dizziness, nausea and feeling enormously exhausted from backpacking into their campsite that they'd made that day. Alison took his friend's vitals. He saw that his blood sugar had skyrocketed. It was so far advanced and their medical supplies so skimpy, it was imperative to get his friend out for emergency treatment. Alison's friend was near death! He was lucky! Alison found a ranger close by who could radio for help. And also, luckily, they hailed a helicopter that was close enough to get his friend to a hospital in time to save his life. Alison's friend was a physician. You'd think a doctor would know better, but he was a neophyte to the trails. He'd only read about backpacking. Heard colleagues talk about it. So, he thought he knew! He was right in thinking he'd need to replenish the energy he'd burn up backpacking. So high-energy bars and alcoholic drinks would be just the thing! But, he'd consumed far too many carbohydrates to replace the energy he assumed he'd burned up on the hike into camp. And he figured, just to be sure not to let his blood sugar level drop too low, he'd have a drink or two before dinner!

It Can't Be Stressed Enough

You need *extra care* for your blood sugar level. This is paramount! For your personal safety. Not too many extra carbohydrates. Nor too few! Don't guess at it. Take along your glucose-monitoring meter. Use it. Use it often.

Hiking is actually good for your diabetes. But you need to play it safe at all times. If I wasn't wise enough to play it safe, and neither was Alison's physician friend, don't you be next at blood sugar roulette! Be sure you carry all your meds, as well as extras. Take along your blood sugar monitoring meter, extra testing supplies, syringes and extra insulin, both types if you are using them. And always carry extra high-energy snacks in your pack. I now watch the energy I spend on short, steep hikes. I've been a diabetic over half my life. And am still learning the consequences if I don't give it full consideration on every hike. I pass this on to you as a serious matter. Better be over-prepared than under-concerned.

Chapter 12

Hiking With a Heart Condition

Can we still enjoy hiking with a heart issue? Not only is it possible. But it can be amazingly enjoyable.

Hiking With Your Heart Issues

The good news is that you can continue to hike even if you've had *serious* heart issues. PROVIDING you take it easy as well as take all appropriate precautions. I am still hiking into my nineties more than fifteen years after open-heart surgery. I've also had an atrial-fibrillation procedure and a few anginas. I'm not a doctor. I am merely telling you what I found works for me. My number one tip is *moderation in all things*. Especially hiking. By all means, if you can walk, you can most likely hike. Even if it's only a few steps along a road. Unless of course your physician says, "No, not you!" Then obviously follow your doctor's advice. And of course, don't take my advice *unless you have an okay from your doctor.* Every one of my doctors urges me to walk, and hike – but always in moderation. There have been a few times that my doctors had me get up onto my feet and walk a few steps down a hospital hall. And they've urged me to walk fifteen minutes every day.

How To Know When to Slow Down

My suggesting you carefully monitor your heart rate while walking is just as important a bit of advice. Regardless of our medical condition, we geezers must give special attention to our heart. Heart attacks are a major cause of death among us old geezers. And heart attacks stalk us with increasing frequency the older we get. Many hiking geezers I know are already carrying their nitroglycerine tablets at the ready. If you haven't done so already, it is wise to speak with your primary care provider if you are *thinking* of going hiking. Even with a cardiac condition, you can probably enjoy a regular daily hike. I speak from my experience of living with cardiac conditions for over twenty-five years. I'm in my nineties and have only slowed down enough to annoy my younger hiking friends. The first, and most critical thing you must do if you've had heart issues, is to see that you don't get another as a result of hiking. And that means keeping your heart rate down to acceptable measures at all times. When you find you're having difficulty breathing, *stop*. Check your heart rate. *If it's the least bit high, wait and rest* until it is back down in a safe range for your age and physical condition. I've learned what to be concerned about as I hike with *my* heart's condition, and how to live with it. You ought to do the same.

Why You Should Know Your Maximum Heart Rate

The faster your pulse, the more stress it puts on your heart. So it is common sense to have this information whatever you are doing. Know your *safe heart rate* for your physical condition at your age. And see to it that you do not allow your pulse to exceed it. Do not exceed it while hiking. Nor mowing the grass. Shoveling snow. Playing tennis. Golfing. Anything at all! *Simply put: do not exceed your safe heart rate during any physical activity.* No matter how young you are, keep your heart rate below your age maximum, adjusted for your physical condition.

How to Calculate Your Tolerable Heart Rate

You can easily find the maximum heart rate for an average person of your age in good physical condition with a simple calculation. Simply subtract your age from the number 220. For someone 65 the age maximum is 155. Subtract 65 from 220. (220 - 65 = 155). Take caution here. *For one number does not fit all.* These heart rates are calculated for people in good physical condition for the calculated age. *This number, 220 less your age, must be adjusted for your physical condition.* The pulse rate of 155 is the maximum for persons 65 years old, *in good physical condition.* Someone hiking a couple of miles a day would be in relatively good physical condition. Still, for maximum safety, it would be best to adjust the "tolerable" heart rate down a notch or two. To be safe I'd suggest about three-quarters of that maximum. So instead of 155, the "tolerable" maximum heart rate would be 116. It would be wiser to stop for a rest either when breathing is noticeably labored or when the pulse reaches 116.

How to Adjust for Your Physical Condition

Here is where it is imperative to be honest with yourself, for this adjustment is subjective. While your doctor can give you guidance, a lot depends on your appraisal of your physical condition. When I had by-pass surgery at 74, I needed to get back *into shape* for any post-op hiking. If I had allowed my heart to reach my age maximum (220 – 74 = 146) immediately after surgery I would probably be dead. So to be safe, I ratcheted my maximum heart rate way down to a beginner's level. No big deal. While recovering, I re-set my personal maximum to half the heart rate for my age. Being 74 at the time, I found the maximum for my age, which was 146. Then I divided that in half, to 73. Thus, on my first hikes after surgery, I stopped hiking when my rate approached 73. (220 – 74 = 146 ÷ 2 = 73). Here is an even easier and more "common sense" gauge for your heart rate. Whenever you begin breathing with difficulty, it is time to stop for a rest. So, after surgery, when my breathing became the least bit difficult, I'd check my heart rate. I wanted to be sure it correlated with the numbers. In other words, I wanted to be sure that my pulse wasn't above 73. *Difficult breathing must always take priority!* Of course, I'd wait until my pulse dropped back down to near my "resting heart rate" before I began walking again. After a few days' walks, when my breathing wasn't labored, and I felt comfortable enough, I'd adjust my tolerable heart rate number up a bit, to about 85. When you are feeling good, and know you are sufficiently physically fit, and your pulse hasn't gone over your adjusted tolerable heart rate, you probably will feel as if you hadn't exerted yourself at all. You may feel well enough to move your max rate up a few points. Raise it cautiously, checking your heart rate at each stage. And be sure it complies with your doctor's advice. These cautions are for your safety. As we age we are dealing with a more delicate and precious instrument. This physical body of ours. It can do wonders for us, if we just take good care of it . . . while we still can.

Personally, with my medics' guidance, I gradually moved my tolerable heart rate, over the weeks, up to seventy-five percent of my age max (220 – 74 x .75 = 109.5). So, my new maximum heart rate was 109.5, rounded off to 110. Again, despite these calculations, I stopped whenever I was huffing and puffing. And I also checked to be sure it wasn't above 110 beats per minute. Always, I wait for my breathing to come back down to near normal before I begin to hike again.

I'm cautious in giving this information because many of us are not as honest with ourselves as we need to be. I am not a doctor. I'm basing this information on American Heart Association recommendations. And I've added my own experience. I'd hate to hear that someone developed a heart condition because of something I said. Remember this, heart disease is among geezers' top three causes of death. So, *be prudent and honest with yourself. And moderation in all things*. If you are honest, you really will know what shape you are in. You are no longer in your twenties. So monitor your heart rate — *honestly.*

How to Adjust Your Maximum for Your Physical Condition

I'm 92 as I write this. At my age the maximum heart rate is 128, a good bit lower than the 146 it was at when I had heart surgery at age 74. Even though I am in relatively good physical condition, I rarely allow my heart rate to reach 128, the top limit for my age, before I stop for a rest. Usually I stop and rest when it hits 110. Or on occasion I'll let it reach 115. It is rare that I allow it to run up to 128, the maximum for my age. That occurs more often when I have just climbed a tough section of trail that used to be a breeze, but not for my age today. Whatever . . . I stop and rest until my pulse drops back down well below 90 before I start hiking again. Those numbers work for me, inasmuch as I'm in fairly good physical condition. In the end, you are the one who needs to judge your physical condition. When in doubt, check with your doctor.

How to Check Your Pulse

Most digital stopwatches have an app for a quick reading of your pulse. Use it if you are comfortable with its accuracy. I'd rather stick with a physical count. After all, I'm dealing with *my* life. So I want the most trustworthy way of checking my pulse. If you can find your pulse on your wrist easily enough, then stick with that. I find it easiest for me to find my pulse by placing my fingertips alongside my esophagus just beneath the chin. It may take a bit of wiggling your fingers around for you to find it. Whatever way you choose to find your pulse, it is wisest to practice finding it at home, before you need to do it on the trail.

Using Monitoring Devices

I've hiked with geezers who've had various kinds of devices to monitor their heart rate. They're fine to use. *If they are accurate*. Be sure to check the pulse registered by the device against a reading with a reliable stopwatch. On occasion I've found that their devices are not accurate.

One friend uses his smart phone with a stopwatch feature. Another has a device he straps to his bare chest to let him know his pulse rate. And two others have smart wristwatches that give them their numbers.

If you are counting your heartbeat, then count it for six seconds. Add a zero for your heart rate. That's the quick measurement. When I want a more precise reading, I count my pulse beat for fifteen seconds and multiply it by four. Of course, the longer the time you count your heart rate, the more accurate the reading. Because this is so important to your life, I'm emphasizing it again. Monitor your heart rate on your hikes. Stop whenever you begin breathing more heavily. Check your pulse. When it reaches your tolerable rate, *stop*. Rest until it returns to normal before hiking again! And, let me go a bit further. Stop hiking *whenever* your breathing becomes heavier, no matter your pulse rate. It's the best way you can help your heart and avoid a heart attack.

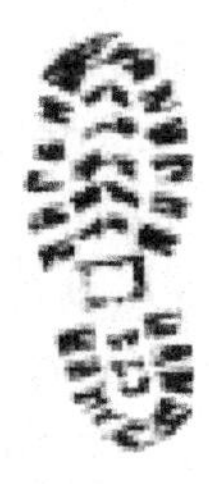

Chapter 13

Correct Your Posture While Hiking

Back in our forties and fifties we never realized how our posture could cause us so many problems as we aged. We didn't know that sitting so much of our day-could cause us such misery and pain as we aged. But the list of our geezering posture problems exceeded the obvious neck, back and butt pains. It's hard to believe the simple things our posture can inflame. Just take a peek at what Harvard Medical School has discovered. Their recent studies connect poor posture with indigestion, constipation and incontinence. (See: https//www.health.health.harvard.edu/staying-healthy/3-surprising-risks-of...) *Who'd have guessed?*

We've also seen even younger geezers bent-over, twisted out of shape. What we don't see is the cruel way their crooked backs are slowly damaging their spinal disks, major blood vessels and especially the nerves that give us those sharp back, hip and leg pains. We also know it's a rare geezer who can just one day *decide* to correct his or her posture. And then succeed. And, of course, the older we get, the more difficult it is for us to change old habits that cause the aggravations. Resolving to correct our posture seems to end like any other New Year's resolution. Lapsed by the third of January! While correcting your posture may not get to its root causes it probably will relieve the pain. And may even cure the ailment. So, if you have neck, back or leg pain, it's always best to start by seeing your doctor. In the meantime, there are some simple posture correction exercises you can do while you hike that will probably relieve most of your pain - improve your overall health and correct your posture.

Must We Live With Pain the Rest of Our Life?

I never did have good posture. And ever since I turned sixty, my posture became more and more senile. Moreover, as I hiked into my eighties, I suffered severe sciatic attacks. They were so painful, persisting without relief, that they prompted thoughts of suicide. My wife wearied of my moaning. So she dragged me to a series of specialists. She took me first, of course, to my personal physician. Then to a kinesiologist. On to a massage therapist. To an acupuncturist. Next a Reiki healer. And so forth. (Surgery was not an option. Two physician hiking friends, one of whom was an orthopedic surgeon, persuaded me to find *any cure at all. But not surgery.* Imagine *that* from a surgeon!) Each specialist gave me relief. And suggested I practice an exercise or two to correct my posture. That was good. But not enough. Then, a stroke of good luck!

My Hiking Companion

While we'd known each other for over a year and become good hiking buds. I hadn't realized Erik's renown. He was a world champion ski racer. Furthermore, I hadn't realized the following either, for we were simply into hiking, but Erik knew a lot about back and leg pains. He'd helped numerous prima donnas world champion skiers with their aches and pains. His career had been coaching world champion downhill ski racers. He was an expert at dealing with ego-sensitive champions. He retired to New Mexico after coaching ski racers to win Olympic gold medals, which really authenticates why he knew that his posture correction tips would work. He coached skiers like Billy Johnson to win the first Olympic goal medal by any male U.S. Alpine skier. And Hilary Lindh to win the first-ever U.S. Junior World championship. After these prima donnas, Backpacker Bill would be a push over! So really, each of Erik's posture-correcting tips were out of a ski champion's handbook. And since his tips worked for me in my late eighties, they will probably work for you.

Posture Correction Therapy

Nor of course, did I have any idea of Erik's therapeutic propensity. Erik ratcheted his hiking pace way down to be with me while I struggled to begin hiking after each of my sciatic episodes. I said "hiking," though we barely "walked" a hundred feet or so those first days. It was all the pain I could endure. Getting out onto a trail with Eric, though, with his encouragement, enabled me ever-so-slowly to increase my daily walking distance a few steps at a time. Lest I minimize this, it took four months of Erik's coaching, for me to resume hiking at something near normal. It was often painfully difficult to begin walking. But by the end of our day's walk I felt so overjoyed I was ready for the next.

Erik's 'Trail-side Manner'

Probably because Erik has been surrounded by physicians his entire life – father, sister, brother-in-law – he was usually hesitant to give advice. And being in a family of doctors, Erik imparted advice gently and judiciously. Despite my having a helpful array of specialists, I attribute my pain-free hiking mostly to Erik's posture correction tips on our daily walks. In fairness, each specialist had urged me to correct my posture. But none were paid for more than an office visit or two. So none could be out on the trails with me a few times a week to aid my rehabilitation.

Erik suggested his tips casually, about one every week or so. His consistency, being with me week after week, was a major part of my recovery, of course. Because of the constraints of writing, I'll have to give you all of his tips at one time. Still, I urge you not to try doing them all at once. Add them to your hikes gradually. Spread them out over a couple of months. Give each tip a week or so of daily hikes before trying the next. Moreover, don't expect a quick cure. Be patient.

Having said that, though, I still think you ought to see results shortly after your first week's attempt. Correcting your posture will give you a much more enjoyable quality of life in your later years.

Erik's Posture Correction Tips

Erik freely gave these tips to me. So I'm freely, too, passing them along to you.

1. *Erik's first tip – thrust your hips forward.*

Thrust your hips forward while you hike, the same as y while skiing. It may feel awkward at first. And e uncomfortable while hiking uphill. But, on the way dowr far more natural. Try this practice on your hikes, daily if pos a week. Get used to it. Thrusting your hips forward tilts your pelvis. When your mind wanders, for it will from time to time. No problem. Simply begin again. And again. And again. Just bring your attention back to your hips each time. And thrust them forward again. Don't give up. If you keep at it, your muscle-memory will take over. It's why Erik gave these practices to me a week or so apart. It gives each one time to become a habit.

2. *Hold your chin up.*

When your chin is up it helps straighten your back. It also relaxes the muscles in your buttocks, which hold the weight of your head if it is tilted forward. When these muscles are taut for long, they give you — don't laugh — a pain in the butt. If your chin is down and your head forward, it hunches your back forward. So, hold your chin up level with the ground. Allow this to be your only practice for a full week. When you forget this practice, not to worry. Just bring it back to mind and pull your chin up. Do this as many times, and for as often, as you need to. Naturally, the hips forward practice will come to mind from time to time. Go ahead, of course, thrust them forward. But, immediately return to your chin up exercise. And try again to give your attention solely to holding your chin up. Do the practice for an entire week. The same as you did with your hips forward practice.

3. *Keep your eyes thirty feet ahead of you*

Keep your eyes on the trail about thirty feet ahead of you. Notice where your chin is when you do this. Your head will tip back slightly, bringing your chin up. This practice is one of the easiest ways to correct your posture while hiking. But, eyes looking that far ahead of you will enable you to see more of what's going on around you. You will be able to see much of where you are stepping by flicking them down from time to time, without moving your head. Try it. See how feels. Your chin will be held up as well. Practice for a week before taking on the next tip.

4. Keep your heels down

Make this more of a mental exercise. Add the practice in a more exaggerated way at the beginning. Start this practice with a little pre-practice to become familiar with an exaggerated version. Step forward and bring the heel down a little hard. And hold it [down] a bit longer as you take the next step. Then [do it with] the other, one after the other, bringing the heels down harder than normal. And hold each down a bit longer. Get the feel of it. Once you get a feel for it, loosen up and hike as you normally would. Keep your heels in mind as you swing your legs forward and come down with your heels just a bit harder than usual. And mentally imagine each heel remaining down ever-so-little-bit longer. Don't try forcing the heel to stay down. Just mentally observe it, imagining the heel remaining a little bit longer.

Another heel practice

Add one more heel practice to give you a focus on your heels. Do this one at rest stops. *Not while hiking*. At a rest stop take hold of a tree with both hands. Stand a couple of feet away from the tree. Now straighten each leg, one after the other. Push down on the heel of the straightened leg with all your weight. Hold it there for a count of three. Do the same with the other leg. Repeat to help the blood and nerve energy flow down the back of the legs to your feet.

5. *Bend your knees slightly as you hike.*

I know, it seems difficult to even imagine doing this. However, the knees are naturally bent as you swing them forward; so try holding them a bit bent as your foot hits down upon the trail's tread. Erik, being a skiing coach, he would-naturally tell me, "Keep your knees bent. *As if* you are skiing." This was the most difficult practice for me. It just seems so awkward. However, it does work. Though difficult.

Give your attention fully to this practice for a week, just as you have with the other four. No worry if your attention slips and slides. Keep trying. You'll get results if you persist. I did. Though when I do it, I still feel like a waddling, bow-legged clown.

6. Pull your shoulders back.

Erik gave me this practice about two months after the fifth tip. He said it is an advanced-level practice. And it is particularly good for both your posture as well as your breathing. Try breathing out through your mouth and emptying your lungs as much as possible. This will cause you to involuntarily inhale deeply after exhaling through your mouth. Like it or not, shoulders back will give you a fine military presence as well. Again, as with the other tips, give it a week's practice with full attention. See what happens.

7. Pull back your chin

This is one more exercise that I really needed. Whenever I spend too much time on my phone – especially texting – my head is bent over my phone unnaturally. The extra strain on the neck gives me what is more commonly called a "text neck." Practicing Erik's tips number two and three to keep my chin up works fine in straightening my back. But I still suffered from "text neck." Chin up, with eyes ahead, did not fully straighten my neck. So I had to resort to a military exercise. After lifting my chin, I pull it back. And I need to see that it stays pulled back while level with the ground.

I now pull in my chin *after* lifting it. But I also try keeping it level with the ground at the same time. Otherwise, my head can be forward with my chin up, making me look like a turkey, which gives me a pain in my back. Sure enough, when I mentioned this to Erik, he said it is another 'advanced' exercise, which he planned to give me next. You need to try it. Pull your chin up. Then *pull it in.*

Try lifting your chin without pulling it in. Then pull it in after lifting it. See if you can feel the difference. Look in the mirror while doing it in each different way. Better still, ask your spouse to tell you the difference. And don't get pissed if she or he laughs.

How To Use These Practices

Take these practices, as Erik gave them to me, a week apart. Practice each one for a week or so before moving on to the next. These tips are not meant to become sweaty workouts. They are mostly mental intentions. Let them become games. I sometimes make one up as I hike to a cadence. Something with a rhythm. I might say to myself one like this: "Hips forward. Shoulders back. Eyes forward. Chin up. And back." These four seem to bring my whole body to a good posture.

I developed muscle memory slowly. After I practiced, one after the other, through the entire list, I rotated practicing them again, one per week. They eventually became habitual. Though I didn't let up. Hopefully my posture is in better shape now than it was. And today, once my posture slips a bit, probably because of my age, I almost immediately feel pains. It is 'red alert' for me to get back to the drill. Within fifty to a hundred yards, focusing upon my posture, going quickly through the whole bevy of Erik's tips, one after the other, I get relief from the pains. If Erik's method corrected the posture of this 93-year-old geezer, it probably can do the same for you.

Find a Good Practice Trail

I found it good to designate one of my easiest trails as my 'posture therapy trail.' I have a one-mile circular path on which I practice these tips. It has a smooth tread. The incline is so gentle that it might as well be in a city park. Consider hiking on a therapy trail as more of a *walk* in a park, than a *hike* on a trail. Mine is convenient, being fifteen minutes from my home. It is perfect for practicing Erik's exercises. I still focus mainly on one exercise per hike. First, I concentrate on thrusting my hips forward. Next day, my chin up. Next, eyes on the trail way ahead of me. And so on, through all seven practices. Then too, taking a week of hiking a mile a day, practicing these exercises one a day, once in a while re-enforces my posture and has done marvels for my entire well-being. You'll be surprised at how easy walking everywhere with a military posture changes so many things in your life for the good. You'll also feel enormously pleased to be pain free.

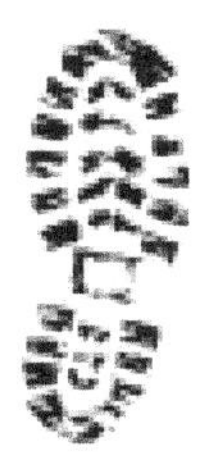

Chapter 14

How to Get Relief from Back Pain While Hiking — Putting the Exercises to Work

I obviously can't diagnose or treat your back pain, for I'm not a doctor. However, the relief I have gotten from a lot of my back pains may be just the trick for you as well. There are simply ways of hiking which I seriously doubt can hurt you, if you do the same. Even if they don't help. Yet none of what I have to say should substitute, in any way, for seeing your doctor if you have back pain.

Relief I Got from My Back Pains

This is really more about how I recovered from some nasty sciatic pains by introducing some simple, easy adjustments to my hiking. They also relieved old back pains I've endured for much of my adult life. They may be useful for you as well, considering I've just learned about them in my nineties and adopted them while still hiking.

The Aging Slump

We naturally begin to slump forward as we age. It's hardly noticeable at first. But without correction there are gloomy times ahead! I know, for I've been there. Twice in two years I suffered severe sciatica attacks that crippled me to the point of considering suicide. I could not cross a room on crutches at the beginning of each episode. Moreover, each time it took me four months to recover well enough to hike on some difficult trails. I'm lucky to have many who helped me through these episodes. Especially my wife, a super-caregiver who encouraged me every day in every way. When I had my last sciatica attack, she was heading out on a three-week trip to Europe with her college roommate. She obviously would not be here for me. She hesitated about leaving me in such a helpless condition. I too, wanted her to go without worrying about me. So, I asked a group of friends for help. It took a good many of them to replace my dear wife. You may feel uncomfortable to ask friends for such help. To be honest, so did I. But there usually is someone who likes to organize things like my friend Damien. He heard my need and quickly jumped to a broader group of my acquaintances and put together a schedule and list for each to take part. To my surprise, there was one or another of them looking in on me every day to be sure I was all right and to get anything I might need. Some days more than one came to see me. They did the grocery shopping and other small chores. Mostly, though, they kept me company for a bit of time each day. And some took me for rehabilitation walks. These rehabilitation walks had begun with my wife, then with these friends, were at first no more than a few hundred feet on crutches. Slowly I began to walk with trekking poles instead of crutches. And gradually I was walking a bit farther on each outing. As I mentioned in the previous chapter, one friend, Erik Steinberg, came two to three times a week for my walks. I was especially lucky to have Erik's friendship. He is a retired US Olympic Ski racing coach who trained skiers to win World Cups in downhill ski racing.

Erik Steinberg's Hiking Backache Therapy

From time to time on our walks, Erik would give me a tip that enabled me to get a bit further along in my recovery. When I followed Erik's advice, I was able to walk for a time without pain. Imagine! Changing habits in my nineties! If I can do it, you probably can as well. I am so grateful to all who helped me, especially Erik, to keep on hiking, which is key to my recovery. Every little bit of help added to my pain free walking.

So here are Erik's simple ways of ridding yourself of most back pains. While these tips were mainly focused on correcting my posture, which of course was the source of many of my pains, they also helped relieve other back pains I'd had for years.

Erik's Five Tips for Pain Free Hiking

1. *Use Hiking Poles*

No matter how slowly you walk or how easy the terrain, there are good reasons to use hiking poles. The most important is that they help prevent falling, and falls are the greatest cause of injuries among geezers, especially back injuries, as I explain in Chapter 8. They also help correct posture, which reduces or even eliminates some back pain, by replacing some of the action your leg muscles use in lifting your feet with each step you take, which subtly reduces stress on those muscles. The poles also enable you to more easily equalize the ambidexterity of your legs, by putting your weak leg forward about an inch while you walk. This reduces pain in the hip and calf of your strong leg, while strengthening the same muscles in your opposite, weaker leg. Proper length of your poles is essential to get relief from this type of pain! They should fit your hands comfortably when your arms are bent at the elbow and your forearms are level with the ground. Actually, you may find them even more effective if your poles are another inch longer than this.

2. *Hike with your hips thrust forward.*

This is Erik's most basic suggestion. He told me, "Try thrusting your hips forward as you walk." He faced me, placed his hands one on each side of my hips and gently pulled them forward. "Feel that? When you push the hips forward like this, you are tilting your pelvis. You are positioning your body directly over your feet. This releases the back muscles from holding your body weight in that off-center position with poor posture. "Can you feel the difference?" It was tilted at the obvious angle my kinesiologist had urged when she'd say, *"Straighten your back."* Excellent advice of course. Though not so easy to do. Erik's tips were just giving me a little bit of emphasis on different parts of my body, making it easier for me to make these changes. Here's another.

3. *Keep your heels down.*

He'd say, "Just focus on your heels as you walk. Keep them down as long as you can without forcing them, as you begin your next step. You will automatically notice your heel staying down as you step forward with your other foot. Just observe them." Oddly enough, I found that walking this way while observing them, each heel, one after the other, tended to stay down a bit longer. And it straightened my back without my even trying.

4. Bend Your knees Slightly as You Walk

As Erik stood up from a trailside bench on which we had been sitting, he bobbed up and down, barely noticeable. He said, "*See my knees*. Like skiing." Try to keep your knees slightly bent all the time you are hiking. It will strengthen the hip maximus muscle. "More important, it will help keep your hips thrust forward, tilting your pelvis. Gives you better balance. And it'll straighten your back, too."

Of course, a major part of my rehabilitation was utilizing these practices on short walks. It would be a while before the walks would be long enough to call 'hikes.' We were walking on a short, mile-long path in the woods. It has a hard-surfaced tread of micro-gravel with very little elevation change. A nice feature is its seven benches spaced out evenly an eighth-of-a-mile apart, providing perfect rest stops. There was little need to be looking down to watch where I was stepping. This even path makes it easy to concentrate my attention on these small practices. I focused attention fully upon my pelvis for one day's walk. My heels on the next. My knees on still another walk. And each week I gave my attention fully to a different one of Erik's backache correction measures. As I write this, I have already practiced each of them numerous times and am making something of a habit of them. And I am now able to hike two to three miles on moderate mountain trails. Erik had more tips.

5. Keep Your Chin Up

Have you ever noticed how many of us old geezer's heads are tilted slightly forward as we walk? It's natural. All the stress that we have borne in our neck over a lifetime has a perfectly natural reaction – a stiff, forward-leaning head. Without correcting this, it literally gives us a pain in the butt. Erik said, "Lift your chin as you walk. And look as far ahead of you on the trail as you can. Hold it up and you will feel the difference in your back. It will release the tension of holding your head forward. And free you of this stress-induced pain." Now, whenever I walk with my chin up level with the ground, I notice I'm relieved of a big part of my irritable butt pain. With all five of these practices, you are bound to have less pain in a short time. Turning these tips into habits will carry over into the rest of your life even when you aren't thinking about them. Most important, it will keep you free of most of your back problems. Since Erik is a frequent hiking partner, he had more to give.

6. Look at the trail as far ahead of you as you can

Keep your eyes on the trail about thirty feet ahead of you. Notice where your chin is when you do this. Bringing your chin up, your head will tip back slightly, holding it directly above your body. By looking thirty feet ahead, your chin will be up, your back straighter and your hips further forward. Each improvement in your posture better aligns your body and head weight directly over your ideal center of gravity. This relieves the stress on thigh, back and butt muscles from carrying excessive amounts of "off-balance" weight. Try it. See how it feels. Obviously, when clambering over roots and rocks, you need to watch more closely where you are stepping. But, keeping your eyes ahead of you and slightly flicking your eyes down without moving your head will allow you to see much of where you are stepping most of the time. Practice this exercise for a week.

This is a good place for me to tell of Erik's best gift of all. I have no doubt it was a big factor in Erik's great success in coaching world champions.

Erik's Sandwiched Critiques

By all means, if you can get a coach like Erik, don't hesitate to bow down to him or her and snatch their advice. Erik explained one day how he managed to tell egotistical champion skiers how to correct something before a big race. Here's how Erik put it: "I couch a critique into a sandwich. "I praise the skier for something he (or she) did well on the run. "Then I tell him the correction he needs to make. "And I follow it by another compliment for his performance. "It softens the correction. And makes it easier for him to make the correction."

These tips will not be as easy for you to make without an Erik to sandwich them for you, as he did for me, but the tips are important to put into practice.

Knee Pull-up

This suggestion comes from my kinesiologist, Karen Zaker. It helps instantly with inexplicable aches, pains and numbness I get from time to time in various parts of my butt and legs. It is *not a cure*. But it seems to send relief in warm energy down from the butt, along the back of the legs to my feet. This is an "extra" exercise. It is no substitute for the other exercises. Nor a substitute for your doctor's advice or for your meds. This tip really just gives us a way to live with some ailments another day. To do the practice, be seated, take one knee with both hands. Get a good grip. Now pull the knee up as tightly to your chest as you can, while pushing your stomach tight to your thigh. Hold it there for a count of ten. Let go and draw up the other knee in the same way, holding it for a count of ten. Repeat this practice as often as you find it useful.

Final Tip. Make Notes to Yourself

This tip is from me. Leave notes in conspicuous places to remind yourself of these particular practices. I carry a half-dozen 3x5 cards in my breast pocket. I jot down notes to myself about anything that pops into my mind during the day that I don't want to forget. These days I often jot one of these tips on a card and slip it onto a slot of the dashboard of my truck where it is conspicuously displayed, It reminds me to do that exercise on the day's hike. Today, for example, I wanted to focus on "chin up." So I jotted "Chin Up" on a 3x5 card, tucked it into a slot of my dashboard. When I got to the trailhead I tucked the card into my pocket. Since I was hiking with someone, it would be difficult to remember to pull my chin up while we chatted along the trail. So, feeling the card in my pocket as I warmed my hand, I'd remember from time to time to lift my chin as we walked. I've done this repeatedly on my hikes. Other days I marked the cards "Hips," or "Heels," or "Knees." I try to work on one small practice a day. I often forget while hiking. But as soon as I recall the day's practice, I get right back into it. And most important, I simply do not allow myself to get discouraged. No matter how often, or for how long, I forget — and I certainly *will* forget – I pick myself up, dust myself off, and start all over again. This is what trails are for me. To get myself back into shape when I have my slips, I just get back to my daily hiking as soon as I am able. Of course, I've developed habits from tricks like these that have kept my hikes a high priority. And I rarely miss a day. If I can do it in my nineties, you may have just as good a chance of refining your hiking habits as well.

Chapter 15

Picking Your Hiking Companions

Whether you are new to hiking, or a seasoned old hand, I've got tips about hiking companions. Hiking alone or with a hiking companion has always been a tricky question. There are as many reasons for going alone as there are for only going with a hiking partner. In the end, it is probably more about personalities. Who you are and who they may be.

If you are new to hiking

I suggest you hike with anyone who'll go with you. At least to get started. After you've been hiking a while, you'll begin to have some options and be able to more carefully discern what it is that you like about other hikers' hiking styles. The need to decide whether to hike with someone before you start hiking with them can become the world's greatest excuse you'll ever need for not going hiking. So take a deep breath, lace up your shoes and get started with whoever shows up. But get started! And with someone more experienced.

So, Rule Number One: Get started hiking! Whether it's with your spouse, siblings, friends, or alone, get outdoors right away and take a walk. Over time you will settle this issue and develop a habit, regardless of who your partner may be.

If You're Reading This Because Of Its Title

You may be in the same boat as I was for many years: loving the trails, but not finding others who love them as much – or at least not in the same way – as you. Like me, you may have tried a dozen or so different companions, and though they are all good people with whom you love doing other things, the trail is not where your compatibilities shine. As we become immersed in hiking, the more we find out about ourselves. Devoid of social constrictions this will help you in choosing your hiking companions. While we are out there in stillness, away from cell phones, computers and television, we begin to truly see our compatibilities, harmonies, discordances and our innermost foibles. We discover that we deeply like some attributes about ourselves, as we also become aware of our ungracious sides. And in the backcountry we learn to accept ourselves for what we are rather than for any falsities of our persona that we put on in our everyday lives back home. Yes, long before we became hikers, we knew we had two selves – one being our social persona built by our nurturing, and the other, truer, deeper, God-given nature. The more we get away from the limiting influences of everyday life, the more we get in tune with this fundamental side of who we are. Our upbringing, no matter how well intentioned our parents, was largely shaped by the word *'don't.'* Don't play with fire; you could get burned! Don't play in the street; you could get hit by a car! Don't be impolite; that's your grandmother who loves you! Don't pick that up off the floor; it's dirty and could have germs! Don't hit your little sister: it's not nice! Don't do this . . . Don't do that . . . On and on . . .

And later in life, the *don'ts* become couched in more genteel-sounding language. Who dresses like that! Not another one of *those!* It's such a relief to be free of other people's ideas of who *we*, or *they*, are. It's the psychological freedom of the outdoors. The more we hike, the more we come to cherish it. And because of this side of our backcountry experience, the more we are out there, the more we want to have around us others like us, who are compatible with our authentic self. So, who we choose as hiking companions becomes critically important. However . . .
The more I hike and the more I find out about myself, the more tolerant I seem to become. I see that others have the same unpleasant character traits as I do, and are just as blind to them as I am to mine. Just knowing this about other people, has enabled me to be far more accepting of them. Nonetheless, I still have my limits. I'm not quite ready yet, for instance, to listen to a companion's self-absorbed political views on a two-hour hike.

So a rule I've followed most of my life is to hike alone. This gave me an ironclad hiking habit that keeps me hiking, rain or shine, heat or snow. Still, if someone wants to hike with me, I'm usually up for it. And if my partner wants to skip a day, I still go on my hike. These days, I'm hiking alone no more than a couple of days a week. I have a mix of people who ask me for a hike, four regulars and my wife. It may be because I am so frightfully slow these days; they know they can hike faster than I can. They are a fine mix. Two are from Texas, one recently from Colorado, and others from back east who've moved out here. Personality-wise, I enjoy their company, though it's very limited with two of them. As long as we are all polite with each other, like most social relationships, we can tolerate each other on an enjoyable hike. Still, I do love my solo hikes on which I can even stop to meditate. Thus I go solo whenever I can, and which I enjoy as much as, if not more than, going with my most compatible hiking companions.

There Will Come a Day

If you depend on a hiking partner, there's going to be a day he or she will not be able to go. Or just not want to go. That will become a perfect excuse for you also to not want to go. And that will be the end of your resolution to take regular hikes. Find a short, easy trail near home where it is safe to hike. Use this trail as a fallback trail on which to take a minimal hike, at times like these. It is best, though, to first hike your "fall-back trail" with someone else from time to time, to get a comfortable feel for it. Then purposely try your darnedest to take a hike on your fallback-trail alone to get a good feel for it. Get so used to it that you know what it is like at various hiking times, in all kinds of weather.

Take more strenuous hikes, of course. And take them in woodlands as close to home as possible. When I lived in New York City, I often hiked in Manhattan's Central Park where trails have a flat, hard, level surface. There are lots of trees and lots of people on the trails. But these paths are fine for a daily hiking (walking) routine. And leave the mountains to weekends and holidays. Well-used trails like these provide a bit of safety. You're less vulnerable than hiking alone in lonely places. I'm not just talking of physical harm, but of accidental injury as well. I have a good friend, for example, a retired tri-athlete, who was injured on a medium-to-difficult mountain hike out here in Northern New Mexico. She severely turned an ankle, coming down on it with all her weight, dislocating her ankle bones. Fortunately, she was hiking with a friend who could go out for help.

It required a litter and two rescuers to carry her out. So, if you choose to hike alone, be sure to prepare for the worst and hope for the best. Foremost, be sure to always leave your hiking plan and the estimated time you expect to be back out with someone reliable. Just in case. And give them instructions of what to do if you are not back out safely at that time. Tell them who to call and what to do next. This may seem like over-kill on beautiful, warm, sunny days. And hopefully, it will be. But, it is far better to be safe than sorry!

Pets on the trail

I always hike with my dog. I've been through a number of these trail companions. They love the trail so much it gives my hikes added pleasure to see them run and sniff the trail. For every pleasure there is a price, of course. Or should I say, "There is no free lunch." It is irritating to encounter a pet out of control on a trail and its owner running after it, trying to make reason out of chaos. On the other hand, there's nothing quite as pleasant as a well-trail-trained dog and its master. I don't mean "master" in a male-gender connotation. A female *master* is something more than "mistress" would imply.

Get your dog trail-trained before you take it hiking. We have a couple of good trainers in town. My wife and I have always gotten our dog's training from a trainer in charge of dogs on our local Search & Rescue Team. A big mistake many owners make is to assume that because their dog will come when called back home it will also come when called on the trail. Bad mistake. They are two entirely different situations for your dog. They have to be trained for the one as strongly as for the other. Another pet annoyance is their scat on the trail. Some of the popular trails have doggy-poop bags available from dispensers at trailheads. It's a hint. Take one or two, and pick up after your dog. It is also a hint to take along a couple of bags on *all* trails. And pick up after Fido wherever he does his business on the trail. If your dog goes far enough off the trail, where no one is likely to step on it, use common sense. No need to become excessive. Most hiking trails in the West permit equestrians, and no one expects them to pick up after their horses. Nor after wild animals that leave their droppings. So your dog can be the ideal trail companion.

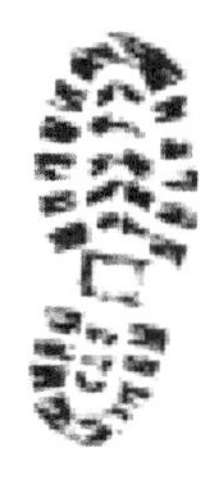

Chapter 16

Hiking Alone

Virtually every 'How-to' hiking book, including my own *Backpacker and Hiker's Handbook,* warns against hiking alone. Yet, here I am, adding a chapter for Geezers on the benefits of hiking alone. So, what's changed? Well, not exactly all, but there are good reasons to think a bit out of the box. The advice is good. Don't go alone until you've got an insatiable need to do so. If the itch so deeply permeates your blood that you just can't resist, then there are some things you ought to do to reduce the higher risk of hiking alone.

Why Many Experienced Hikers Hike Alone

I don't know a single highly experienced hiker who doesn't hike solo from time to time. Here's Denise Traver, for instance, a backpacking trip leader at the Grand Canyon, who seems something of a zealot solo hiker. Between guiding trips, Denise takes extended treks alone. She says, "Solo hiking is addictive. It opens my eyes to the unbelievable beauty surrounding me when I am off by myself. "I took my first solo backpacking trip for six days into the Superstition Mountains near Phoenix and haven't looked back since." That's excessive for most of us. However, her reasons seem the same for most of us getting off on solo hikes. At least they are for me. When I'm with others, I'm unable to just sit beneath a leafy tree and immerse myself so intently into the stillness and relax that I'll actually hear falling leaves touch down upon other leaves on the ground. And I agree with Denise that solo hiking is addictive. It seems the more I do, the more I want to hike by myself. The stillness is overwhelming. While I love chatting with a hiking friend, it stands in sharp contrast to what I see and feel when I am alone — the stream's burble, seeing a rare dark-crested stellar jay hopping through the brush, a solitary twitter of an unidentified bird. And just feeling a soft summer breeze on my cheek. I'd say all of the forest is far more intense when I am by myself. And more relaxing. No doubt this is why Japanese physicians now prescribe solitary forest visits for high-strung patients.

How to Start Solo Hiking – As Safely As Possible

Before you take a single solo hike, be sure to read ***all*** of my cautions of the heightened risks of hiking alone. While hiking alone is riskier than hiking with a partner, these do's and don'ts will reduce those risks substantially.

1. *What to Carry in Your Pack*

I'm presuming you are already an experienced hiker. At least you should be, to even consider hiking alone. So, you will already know what to carry in your pack. However, I advise you to take another look, just to be sure not to omit anything. There's no one from whom to borrow an extra high-energy bar. So, I strongly advise that you go to REI's Check List and give it a considerable amount of attention. It's the most exhaustive list I'm aware of. It is excessive on purpose. For depending upon where you live and the time of year you will need certain items that are extra baggage elsewhere. (See: https://www.rei.com/learn/expert-advice/day-hiking-checklist.html) In the beginning don't hesitate to go overboard in what you take. You can always pare it back as you become more experienced.

2. *Begin small.*

Start with hikes of no more than an hour or so. Start by forming the habit of turning back after you've hiked about thirty minutes. Build a bit longer time on that as you become more confident and comfortable with other hikers on the trail.

3. *Pick your trail wisely*

Hike solo only on busy trails at times when there are sure to be other hikers. Actually, if you were to hike on any of the busier trails around here you will see many solo hikers, as if they were just out for a Sunday stroll. If you were to hike any day on a trail I've frequented the most in the past several years, for instance, you'd see that well over half the daily hikers are hiking alone. Unlike Denise's six-day backpacking jaunts, though, I'm talking about daily hikers. On the first three or four miles of this trail. Should you decide to take your first solo hike, this would be the sort of busy trail that would be safest for you to try.

4. Know your ability and comfort level

Be sure to take a trail that's well within your comfort level. Be sure the trail is well-marked, and well-maintained, and that there is no chance of you getting lost. The best trail would be one that you have hiked before with a hiking partner. And its difficulty level should be well below the limit of your hiking ability. Do not take a trail with higher difficulties like stream crossings, exposure, dense un-cleared brush, anything that has a higher risk. While you should obviously reduce risks of accidents, should you nonetheless have an accident or health emergency you'd welcome other hikers who could at least call or go out for help.

5. Stay on the trail.

Carry as detailed a map of the trail as possible. And be sure to follow trail markers. If there are any trail junctions, it's good to take a picture of them, if possible. Or, see that there is clear signage indicating directions you fully understand. It's important to recognize them properly on your return. For they will not look the same on your return. I was shocked on a recent hike I took with two highly experienced hikers. We'd stopped for a rest and were into some captivating conversation. When we started to hike again, we headed in the wrong direction. While I suggested we were making a mistake, they even persuaded me to head in the wrong direction. It was on a level stretch of nondescript tread. We continued our hike deeply engrossed in our chat, when finally we came upon an obvious landmark outcropping. One of our "experts" noted that there was something wrong, that this outcropping should be on the other side of the trail. And then, WHOOPS, almost unanimously we all realized we were heading "out" and not "back" on the trail. It can happen to the best of us. So, extra caution!

6. Check the weather forecast.

While you may like hiking in rain or snow, it is safest to take your first solo hikes on clear days. So get a weather forecast before you step out onto the trail. Where I live, the weather in summer can change rapidly in the afternoon, making mountain hiking especially dangerous because of lightning. Furthermore, the trail tread can become dangerously slippery when wet.

7. Leave information about where you'll go and when you'll return

Tell someone reliable where you are going, when you expect to be back and what to do if you aren't back then. I probably ought to have made this the first precaution, it's so important. This is especially important for all solo hikes. But, I'd say, even more important for your first ones. If you are within wireless range be sure to text your contact before and after your hike.

*8. Do **not** wear headphones.*

There are just too many sounds that can suddenly be an alert – a sudden change in weather, a shout from another hiker, an animal. The possibilities are almost endless. I've been alerted from spooking a rattler on our road, the least likely place I'd expect one. It might have struck me, had I been wearing headphones and not heard its warning rattle.

9. Know your limits

Be sure you honestly know your comfort level and try to remain well within it. Be sure you are not pressing your limit before turning back. It's no time to see how far, or fast, you can hike. Don't. Please do ***not*** - see how much you can do at your age. Dropping dead on a trail may sound romantic, but consider the years of pleasure that can still be yours inasmuch as you are in good enough shape to be hiking. No matter your age, you must know that many others are no longer with us.

10. Know you local wildlife

Know the likelihood of encountering a bear or snake. And what to do about it. This information is readily available at your local outfitting shop. Or from other hikers. Don't become overly concerned. Just be aware. And prepared.

11. Trust your instincts

If something doesn't feel right, it probably isn't. Know yourself well enough that you know what and how to take care of yourself. Trust your instincts. Better be wrong and safe, than the alternative!

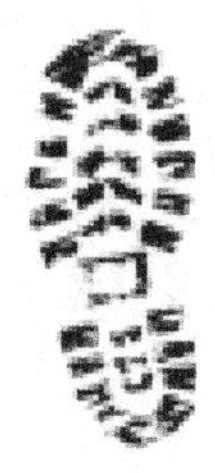

Chapter 17

Why I Still Keep Hiking Into My Nineties

As an old geezer, I of course have different reasons today for hiking than I did at nineteen. You may share my reasons, even if you had to stay away from the trails for years because of your career. Or maybe you've dabbled in the outdoors, but now want to give it a go in your retirement.

Love of the Woods

You likely share some of my love of the outdoors that I still have from my earliest years. No matter what your physical condition, it's quite possible that you can get into hiking. It isn't particularly difficult. Actually, if you can walk you can hike. Hiking is so easy that even I, who am not at all athletic, can hike. I love its benefits so much that I take every opportunity to at least saunter on a walk wherever I am.

Let me share one of those love-of-the-woods moments from my early adulthood. I'd been away from trails for the years I served in the military and the first years of college. Even without a car at college, though, I took walks in New York's Central Park and Riverside Park, which runs along the Hudson River just a block from where I lived near Columbia University.

One day, when I finally had a car, I drove up to the Catskills, parked in the campground at the end of Woodland Valley Road and got out of my car. I was overcome with so much joy that I threw up my arms and shouted, "God, thank you! *Thank you* for bringing me back. Why, oh why, have I stayed away so long?" I was not embarrassed over my outburst, for there were no others there. The campground was usually empty back in the 1940s. I did not know another hiker in those years. I have been hiking or walking for a lifetime, and have continued hiking on into retirement at sixty-five. And I am still at it in my nineties. And most of my "hikes" are sauntering on easy trails.

Here Are Ten Reasons Why You Too Can Enjoy Hiking

1. *First is foremost.* The joy of hiking helps get my butt out the door on chilly days when I feel that the fireplace is more appealing.
2. *It's easy to hike no matter what my physical condition.*
3. *It's good for my heart and my health.*
4. *I can walk when I cannot hike.* I can walk virtually any place I happen to be whether city or country, near a trail or only a sidewalk.
5. *The only equipment I need is a comfortable pair of shoes.* When I begin to hike a rougher trail, a pair of sneakers suffices. However, using trekking poles to prevent falling is well worth the price.
6. *I do not need a partner.* I can hike alone if I use common sense where and how far I hike.
7. *It's inexpensive.* There are almost endless places that are free to hike.
8. It relieves my mind of useless worries. I find hiking makes it difficult, if not impossible, while on a trail, to keep my mind on things that trouble me back home.
9. *It is a good place to be close to God.* Next to cathedrals and scripture it's compelling for me to feel reverence while in the woods.
10. *I find it easy to meditate while hiking.* While there is an ancient Burmese Buddhist walking meditation I learned back in my twenties, I prefer to stop for a rest and meditate seated for fifteen minutes or so. The peacefulness of the woodlands is just perfect for it.

All in all, I cannot be on a trail more than fifteen minutes before I lose all sense of the city. It is best when I am by myself. It isn't just being out there; I am speaking of being alone. I find it a privilege to hike with friends who are good company, but it nonetheless distracts. My hiking companion requires my attention. Rightfully so, for I truly am sociable. Then too, while three is a crowd, I'm horrified to see or be with groups out on a trail. No matter how small and quiet a group, it just takes the wild out of wilderness. Nonetheless, if you need company to hike, by all means hike with others rather than not hike at all.

Clearly Each Of Our Days Are Numbered

I know my end is near. And I'm getting wobblier by the day. I've had a series of health issues, one after another in the past six months. For I'm getting into what you might say is a more "limited" condition. Still, I'll be darned if I want to become so limited I can't take my hikes, even if they are just around the corridors of a hospital. So as I have said, keep on hiking the best way possible. That is, if you want to enjoy your last few days as much as I'm enjoying mine. At whatever age and condition, you never know what is going to happen in the next fifteen minutes! Sure, I'm being a bit extreme, but it is such an integral part of my life that my walking and hiking are major reasons that keep me going.

We No Longer Need to Set Records

I no longer am out there to accomplish anything at all on a trail. I don't see how far or how fast I can hike. I don't need to hike to any special place to see something special. For years it's been enough to only want to see what's over the next hill or around the next bend in the trail. If you've read this far you most likely have similar inclinations. Or perhaps you want try find a way to help someone else get out on the trails. No problem. I've hiked, camped, and played outdoors for the lion's share of my life. In fact, I've hiked several times every year, except for the time in the Navy and while at university without a car.

Hospitalization Does Not Have to Stop You From Hiking

Let me tell you about a really easy walk that I took when others much younger than I wouldn't try it. Yes, I recently spent five days in the hospital. While there, I hiked the halls of the cardiac unit of the Raymond G. Murphy VA Hospital in Albuquerque. I was recovering from another "possible" heart attack. I would have gone stir crazy if I had to spend those five days lying in a hospital bed. So of course, all day long and much of the night, I trod a circuit around and around through the halls. It didn't get as boring as my stay would have been had I been confined to my room.

They dubbed me "the Wanderer"

I probably wandered a couple of miles a day through those halls. Even when I was attached to an intravenous bag, the other end hanging from what they called "a Christmas Tree," I simply rolled the tree along beside me.

Getting to Know the Staff

I kept passing hospital staff – doctors, nurses, nurses assistants, clericals, meal deliverers, clean-up chums and some I never figured out what their job was, though they were all busy bees. They got to know me. And I got to know them – a lot better than had they just brought me my meds and shots. One fellow, Steve Ifill, during a slack period late at night, took me walking. They had a GPS instrument fastened to my chest to keep track of my whereabouts. So Steve had to get permission to take me off limits to explore secret passages of this massive hospital.

Patience for Other Patients

I've got to say, these women and men put in tough shifts taking care of us patients. At the peak of my five-day stay, there were sixteen men and two women patients. Most of them needed a lot more attention, though I was easily fifteen to twenty years older than most. Some took falls and had to be picked up and cleaned up. Some were much more serious cardiac trauma cases. But most of the patients, at some point, were ambulatory and urged to get out of bed and take a walk – "like The Wanderer."

Why Do I Keep on Hiking Into My Nineties?

I hike because of my deep love of nature, of course. You probably love the woods as well. The Japanese have found that most of us have this affinity for the forests. They scientifically discovered, for example, that there are great health benefits from simply being out among the trees. And that may explain why we enjoy spending time outdoors, meandering among trees beneath an open sky. You also may find it just as re-invigorating. But then, I just feel *better outdoors* – even on the crowded streets of New York City where I lived for years. And there is nothing shabby about a walk in Central Park on a Sunday afternoon. Though of course, I did prefer the woods and brooks of New York's Catskill Mountains.

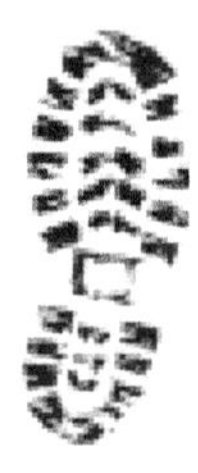

Chapter 18

All-Season Hiking - On Into Winter

I might have said "*Spring* hiking" or "*Autumn* hiking." So why "*On Into Winter*?" Snow! Ice! Cold! They're obvious obstacles.

Not counting the West Coast and Deep South, most Americans know winter snows. Except for bugs, however, hiking in spring and fall is much the same as in summer. The spring does have more bugs; while the fall is pretty much bug free. And of course, so is winter. I encourage geezers to continue hiking, of course, in spring and fall. But hike also in winter, regardless of cold, snow and ice.

I was out hiking a couple of days ago, as I write this chapter, and had to slow down to a crawl in twelve to fifteen inches of new fallen snow. I couldn't hike as far as normal, of course. However, most of the winter has been far easier treading the trails, mostly in boot grippers for packed snow and icy patches.

In fact, I love winter hiking, as much if not more, than I do summer hikes. For one, there are fewer hikers on the trails, giving me more of the peace and solitude I love so much. And two, because the trees are magnificently beautiful laden with snow. A lot of long-time hikers know what I mean, for they're on the trails in the dead of winter as well. Of course, better not to take your first hike in the winter, unless it'll be on a warm sunny day in Florida or Southern California. It would also be wise to go with someone more experienced in winter hiking to give you tips for warmth and safety.

But with a little preparation and a few more items of gear, you can easily shift into an all-season hiker.

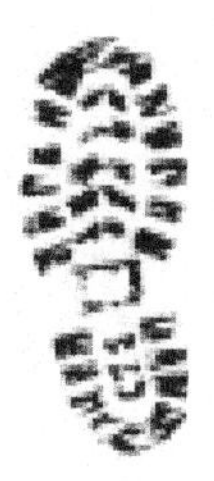

Chapter 19

Geezer Backpacking

Of the miles and miles of hiking I've done, I've loved the backpacking ones best. It's hard to beat sitting at a campfire into the wee hours. Though I do find it just as pleasing to wake up with the birds at first light of dawn. Of course, I often nuzzle back down in my sleeping bag for just a few more winks. Much of my geezer backpacking has been as enjoyable as it was in my younger days. I was ninety when I hung up my backpack for good. I'd gone on a four-day backpack with my youngest brother. We'd gone down into the Rio Grande Gorge to a hidden lean-to I knew about. It's right there on a busy trail, down next to the river. But barely more than a couple of locals know about it. It is hidden behind a thick grove of pine and brush. We hadn't hiked together for over twenty years – he in Vermont, me living in New Mexico. Somehow we'd both mellowed so that we were a continual howl the whole trip. Afterwards, when I thanked Mike for such a good time, I added that it was absolutely the most enjoyable backpacking I had ever done. He joined in with "Likewise." I told Mike it had pushed my limits and I'd decided to hang up my pack after such a great, unbeatable trip. Thus far, I've stuck to my resolution, with not a flicker of temptation to deviate. From time to time, after I became a geezer, I've had to make some creative adjustments to my backpacking because of circumstances. In fact, these 'adjustments' often improved my hikes more than they compromised them.

I've loosely sorted a few treks according to 'adjustments.' I've put them into seven categories. Sometimes I've had to make more than one adjustment to a hike. I am very flexible in how I modify them. The real reason I'm hiking is to be outdoors.

Here are seven examples of hikes to which I've made 'adjustments' to my backpacking during my geezerhood. I hope they give you ideas that make your own hikes as enjoyable as mine have been for me.

1. *Modify your plans for unforeseen circumstances.*
2. *Lighten your pack and shorten the distances.*
3. *Set up a trailhead camp.*
4. *Go car camping and day-hike from the car.*
5. *Get a younger hiker to carry some of your load.*
6. *Set up a base camp and day-hike from there.*
7. *Shuttle gear into a campsite on two or more trips.*

The Adjustments

1. *Modify your plans for unforeseen circumstances.*

My backpacking after 65 has often been modified, though the modifications usually turn out to make our hike "the way to go." A good example is when my daughter, Katie, took me to Europe for an eightieth birthday present. She said, "You always wanted to take us on a hike around Mont Blanc, Dad. But we never got to it. So I want you to take that hike before it's too late."

When we arrived in Chamonix, we discovered that due to late winter snows, some of the lifts and a couple of high mountain huts were closed. That was a crushing blow to Katie! She'd taken such care in arranging everything to give her 80-year-old dad the hike of his life. So, we mourned our loss for an entire day.

On a trial hike the day before we were to get started, Katie got a bad hitch in her back from her pack. And after a day with my load, I realized that I was going to become more of a burden than what we'd anticipated. So, we reshuffled the deck.

We ended up hiking just as many days as we would have with our original plan. But instead of staying every night in high mountain huts, we would take a lift back down to town, stay in an inn where we'd have left our gear. Then, we'd take a lift back up to the route in the morning and continue our hike to another lift where we could ride back down to town. We were usually back down in town by late afternoon in time for a gelato. Later in the evening, we'd dress our best to have dinner at a stellar restaurant. We took most of our hikes on either the north or south side of the mountain where there were the most lifts. Thus, we could stay a few nights at the same inn in Chamonix on the French side, or in Courmayeur on the Italian side. This gave us the option of eating in whichever of their fine restaurants we chose.

There were a couple of segments where we ate lunch in a mountain hut and were so attracted to it that we lingered longer. And we hiked back to and from it to have lunch. After all, we had time, inasmuch as we'd given up our more rigid original plan. While we couldn't have made it around the entire mountain route because of the closures, we turned our ten days of hikes into perhaps an even greater pleasure! A hiking lemon into lemonade?

2. Lighten your pack and shorten the distances.

My nephew, Kenn, and I have a special love of the Grand Canyon. We've hiked there so often, we've covered nearly all the mapped trails as well as a number of off-trail routes. The canyon is deep and takes several days to get in and back out of prize areas. That means the greatest amount of travel and the least amount of time for good backpacking. So, as we became geezers, Kenn and I drew up a system that reversed the numbers. It gave us as much pleasure on a four-day weekend as we'd had on much longer hikes.

Kenn and I each live an equidistance from the Grand Canyon – he in California and I in New Mexico. So it's a nice place to meet after a day's drive each. For a number of years, we put in splendid, relaxed, three-day hikes down in the Grand Canyon for just a day's travel each way to and from the canyon.

Once, when my itch arose for a Grand Canyon hike, I called Kenn. He was sorry, but didn't think he could get away. So, I went anyway. I arrived about 10 P.M., got a room and dropped off to sleep with my alarm set for an early rise. Sometime deep in the night, there was a pounding on my door. I couldn't imagine! Fire? Earthquake? What? More pounding and, "Uncle Bill! Uncle Bill!"

"Who?" I said groggily.

"It's me, Kenny. I'm here."

"You're *what*?"

This was before cell phones. Kenn had no way of letting me know that he was able to get loose after all.

He'd called me at home shortly after I'd left. My wife, Joy, told him where I planned to stay that night. And now, there was Kenn at 3 in the morning. We had time for a two nights' hike. We weren't particularly fussy, as we realized how difficult it would be to get a permit. They're almost impossible to get without applying months in advance. We were in luck to get an "at-large" camping permit cancellation for a not very exciting area. So okay, we were in no position to be choosy.

We started down a heavily used trail, soon found an unlikely place where we could hike off-trail a piece. There are rules about where you may camp. Well, we found an unfound spot, clear enough of cactus and rock, wide enough to make camp atop a rise between two arroyos. But it was nicely hidden from the trail, tucked behind some good-size boulders. And about a twenty-minute hike to a water source. After we got used to our camp, we began to realize how outstanding it turned out to be. It had amazing views, especially as the sun broke above the canyon rim in the morning! Actually, I don't think you can find *any place* in the canyon that doesn't have spectacular views. And our little gem had its share. We stayed our allotted time and knew we'd be back. Its major attraction was that the location enabled us to hike to it in about two hours from our car.

After that, we'd frequently meet at the canyon for a four-day hike, using our secret, hidden, primitive campsite. It also kept our pack weight light. We only needed to carry our sleeping bag, one ground tarp for the two of us, a thin rubber mattress apiece, rain parka, light-weight MSR stove with fuel enough for two days, a pot, a cup, a bowl, and utensils apiece. Plus, food as well as lightweight pullovers for cool evenings. Probably no more pack weight than about twelve to fifteen pounds each.

3. Set up a trailhead camp.

While climbing Colorado's fourteeners, I had discovered car camping was *de rigueur* for Colorado peak baggers. However, since fourteeners are something of a sweat, I'm only suggesting peak-bagging for geezers on the younger side. But, I am recommending overnighting at trailheads for day hiking in to the backcountry. Virtually any National Forest provides an endless number of USFS roads for this opportunity.

One of the best fourteeners I climbed was from a camp that Steve Bridgehouse and I made less than a mile from our car at the confluence of two mountain streams. Steve and I had become friends when he was a Grand Canyon backcountry ranger in the years when Kenn and I hiked in the canyon a few times each year. At the end of Steve's day, we'd often get together to chat over coffee in the Bright Angel Lodge. Steve always spoke of his desire to do some Rocky Mountain climbing. So, eventually, he and I headed into Colorado's San Juan Mountain Range for a peak climbing two-some, Uncompahgre and the more difficult Wetterhorn.

We took on Uncompahgre first, the easier of the two peaks. It was a gorgeous day and we reached the summit just before noon, finding the last fifteen to twenty feet of the climb the most thrilling as it steepens and requires some strenuous moves to the summit.

Back at camp, we began studying the route up Wetterhorn, eye-balling it from camp. The summit ridge, which the trail apparently traverses, still seemed deep in snow. We did not have crampons or ice axes. We questioned whether it would be wise to attempt the climb. "So, Steve, maybe another day?"

"No problem," he said. "We've had two great days already. Just backpacking into this campsite and crowning Uncompahgre. And in good company! So, yeah, let's not push it." I liked that. Bravo. We opted for caution.

4. Go car camping and day-hike from the car.

I turned to car camping and day-hiking on some of my most memorable trips with my father as he passed his seventieth year. I gave him a backcountry trip for his seventieth birthday. We went to Death Valley and car camped out under the stars at various locations from a spot below sea level, to a campground near Stovepipe Wells, to various other primitive camping spots, our last at ten thousand feet high in the mountains next to the valley. We enjoyed ourselves so much that I gave him a backcountry trip every year for the next ten years, right up into his eighties. One of our earliest was a car camping jaunt in Canyonlands National Park. It was still wild back then, in the late 1970s and early 1980s — the days of Ed Abbey's *Desert Solitaire*. Few people yet knew the possibilities of trekking among these weird, twisted, rust-colored sandstone spires. We rented a Jeep in Salt Lake City, filled it with jugs of water, groceries for a week and a full tank of gas and headed south to Canyonlands. Once there, we took a major four-wheeling trek on the White Rim Road, which winds 100 miles around Island In the Sky Mountain in the park's interior. We drove for three days atop the ledge-rock shelving, sleeping nights under the stars next to our Jeep. We drove ever-so-slowly; stopping often to take exploratory hikes. It was delightful to sink so comfortably into the quiet rhythm of the desert. At Dad's age and physical condition, it made for perfect wilderness trekking.

We got to know each other more as men, than as father and son. That was a bit of a surprise for both of us. Unfortunately, those days are gone now. Dad passed away in his early eighties. And much of the "wilderness" of those days is also gone. But, I have rich memories that I'm revisiting in this chapter of my book.

5. Get a younger hiker to carry some of your load.

The idea of spending a few days on a trail with my youngest brother, Mike, was far more exciting than hurting my ego by not carrying all of my share of the pack weight! Mike and I hadn't hiked together for over twenty years. The idea had my juices flowing. Considering my age, this might be the last opportunity I would have to spend this sort of time with Mike. It was generous of him to jump so quickly at my invitation. And come all the way over from Vermont. Just for a hike.

So, just as soon as Mike arrived, we headed straight to the trailhead. I had our gear already in the truck. We arrived at Wild Rivers with enough time to set up camp, build a fire and eat dinner before dark.

The Usual Dis-comforts of Camp Life

It was at this point that Mike and I began to notice things that, in my haste to get onto the trail, I had forgotten to bring along. The first missing item was a second pad to put beneath our sleeping bags. We were camping on a tarp spread out on the ground. Since I sleep well on hard surfaces, I slept in my sleeping bag on the bare tarp. This was only the beginning. I should have titled this section the 'The *Mis*-Comforts of Camp Life' instead of the '*Dis*-Comforts.' It began, as I said, with the forgotten sleeping pad. Not so bad. But others were.

For one, we had no idea the nasty no-see-ums would be so bad. We slept under the stars that first night. Then we slept down at a lean-to situated on the banks of the Rio Grande. Nights were warm enough that we slept half-in and half-out of our sleeping bags. The no-see-ums had a feast on our ankles, arms, faces and necks. I also failed to bring sunscreen. And of course, at our higher altitude the sunrays are intense. Other forgotten items like paper towels and my cigars were nuisances, but not so uncomfortable.

However, not bringing along our first aid kit became a problem. I fell twice on the hike. On one fall I scraped my arm against rough rock surface. And of course, we had no Band-Aids to stop the bleeding. Now we realized I forgot to bring the first-aid kit. Fortunately, Mike has done a good amount of time in an EMS unit. And he has a good sense of making-do with what you have. So he wrapped a makeshift padding of Kleenex tying it in place with a strap from my sleeping bag roll.

Mike and I were in no hurry to go anywhere. But, we actually did take some hikes in between chats around our campfire. Our longest hike was over to Big Arsenic Spring where we stopped for lunch. Then we hiked a little beyond to some distinct Indian petroglyphs. And of course, we hiked back to our lean-to. I doubt, all told, that we hiked more than a good five miles during our stay down there. And of course we hiked the few miles in and out.

All sorts of habits we have in common made it easier to read each other's moods and inclinations so that things just ran more smoothly with us. It certainly added to Mike saying later that it was the best hike he'd ever taken. And I have much the same feelings, which have a special significance for me. I've been so fortunate to have the most magnificent life in the outdoors. Wouldn't it be wise to cap it off with the best? And this *was the best!*

6. Set up a base camp and day-hike from there.

The first geezer backpacking compromise I made turned into one of the most enjoyable hikes I've ever taken. My nephew, Kenn, and I wanted to explore an Arizona wilderness area that is only sixty air miles from Phoenix. Aravaipa's narrow, twisting eleven-mile stretch of wilderness canyon winds through abundant groves of cottonwoods. Water flows into it from seeps, springs and side canyon tributaries. The actual wilderness extends well up and beyond the canyon out onto surrounding ledges, caves and tablelands. It also is a flyway for over two hundred species of birds. Hiking is limited to fifty a day. And backpacking is limited to two nights per visit.

We considered backpacking from one end to the other. However, with a little map study, we saw that it would require far too much highway driving to spot a vehicle at each end to allow us to retrieve one vehicle after backpacking through the canyon. So we worked up an alternate adjustment. We decided to backpack in and out from one end, instead of hiking one way all the way through. We drove one vehicle from Tucson to the remote end of the canyon and camped just outside the canyon our first night. Early next morning we backpacked in as far as we could and set up a base camp for our entire time in the canyon. We each had obtained a two-night permit. One was for two nights following the other's two, giving us four nights all together. Hence, we had one day backpacking in and one carrying out. But three full days hiking farther in, exploring side canyons at our leisure, without having to set up and take down our camp every day. That turned out to be far more enjoyable than it could ever have been backpacking through the canyon. And it gave us different perspectives on how we might go on our next backpacking trips.

7. Shuttle gear into a campsite on two or more trips.

Kenn and his wife, Cheryl Kelly, live on a ranch in Ramona, California. When I visit, they often take me on a drive across the mountains to the Anza-Borrego Desert just east of them, which are a great treat for me. This is where Kenn and I refined our fine art of geezer backpacking. He was becoming more limited with Parkinson's and my age was working its thing on me, so we both needed to slow down a bit.

We rarely camp in campgrounds. There are always too many people and lots of noise of RV generators and bothersome others' comings and goings. So, when we'd arrive in Anza-Borrego, we'd stop for an ice cream, then cruise the blacktop into the heart of the desert until we'd scope out a perfect camping spot. It would have to be a good distance from the road since driving off-road anywhere was prohibited. Once we picked our 'perfect campsite', we'd begin lugging our gear into it. I use the term 'lug' for it really didn't look as if we were backpacking. Of course, our sleeping gear and tent had to be carried in backpacks. And then a second backpacking trip was needed for carrying food and cooking gear. Then, too, there were several jugs of water to bring in to camp. Our campsites were always a half- to three-quarters of a mile away from the car. It usually took us a couple of hours to set up camp, then we'd sit for a couple of hours with a cool drink from the ice chest, admiring the remote setting of our campsite. We'd camp for three or four nights in the same location. During the cooler part of the day, we'd go for a hike at some fascinating spot.

Much of the draw of the Anza-Borrego Desert is the archival remains of Ancient cultures. We took several relatively short day hikes including some to well-preserved pictographs.

Ghost Mountain Trail

One hike, which we took a few times, was to Ghost Mountain and the remains of the home of a desert-dwelling author, Marshal South, with his wife, Tanya, and their three children. Why hike the mile, 1200-feet elevation gain, to Ghost Mountain more than once? It was our fascination with this family living in such austere conditions during sixteen years from 1930 to 1946, through the years of the Great Depression and World War II.

Marshal South was one of the pseudonyms he used during the course of a life hiding from various characters, beginning in childhood fleeing from a rich and dangerous father. The flight to the desert was mainly to be free from city living expenses. He wanted to adopt the life of Native Americans, living mainly off the land, supporting his family with the meager income of a poet, artist, author of articles, short stories and novels. His wife, too, was a poet and artist. His principal income was from *Desert Magazine*, which published his stories, poems and accounts of his family's desert life. He developed a large following, many of whom came to the desert to visit and who sent gifts for Christmas, mainly for his children.

The most fascinating aspect of their desert abode was that they hauled everything that they used, including water, a mile up to the 1200-foot mountaintop. It took twelve gallons of water a day until they constructed a cistern to catch rainwater. At their peak, fifty or more visitors came each year. To discourage visits, Marshal had his family become nudists.

Climbing just once up their steep path made us humbly admire Marshal's continuous feats of carrying awkward, heavy building materials and supplies up that path. And how he managed somehow to carry it all up there mainly on his own shoulders. The children were far too young to help. And his wife was fully occupied with a few loads on top of caring for the children and the household. He hauled up an enormous number of bags of cement to build their house and an outdoor oven. Never mind hauling up their household furnishings, bags of seed and grains, canned food and especially water!

Other hikes had a variety of interest. There was the Mortero Trail, for instance. It's a short hike to an area once inhabited by Kumeyaay Indians. They had carved large morteros, or grinding bowls, into large boulders. They used these morteros over 2,000 years ago to grind local nuts and seeds into meal.

The Motel Alternative

Obviously, we might have chosen to stay in a desert motel instead of lugging our gear into a desert retreat. It would have given us considerably more comfortable sleeping. But we would have missed what Kenn and I love most, the 'feel' of the desert. Should I tell you of our most adventurous relationship to the Anza-Borrego desert? It is a true story.

One evening, just before dark, we were sitting in our camp chairs sipping our hot chocolate, when we had an uninvited camp visitor. You probably guessed it. We had a three-foot long rattlesnake amble its way slowly across our bow. We had to remove it a 'safe' distance away from camp. But he'd left its mark, making it less comfortable going to sleep knowing we might have such night visitors. Were I to cleanse this book completely, it wouldn't leave you with the right flavor of the backcountry. The snake was no harm to us. It made us a bit more understanding of what needed doing to make ourselves more comfortable out there.

Just keep vigilant as you hike. And realize that rattlesnakes are far more frightened of you than you are of them. Our Anza-Borrego rattler would have turned away from our sleeping area and been no trouble for us. It was good to have seen it when we did, in the daylight. Rather than see it at night when one of us got up to take a whiz!

Conclusion

Now you know what to do and why. You know the rewards of hiking, its many joys and tribulations. You know how to do it; how to proceed every step of the way. You know the obstacles to overcome and the excuses you'll tell yourself. But you also have a plan.

So, which will it be? A longer, healthier life full of joy and the wonder of nature? Or a quick decline into boot-less-ness?

The path ahead is clear; the choice is yours. The fraternity of geezer hikers welcomes you with open arms and clear, if sometimes halting, strides. For inspiration you might want to *think* Grandma Gatewood. After raising eleven children, Emma Gatewood wanted to be alone. So, at 67, never having hiked before and despite her age, she hiked the entire 2000-mile A.T. alone. Furthermore, she hiked its length again — twice more before she was 77!

Embrace the choice and see the world open to you with a sense of purpose, rekindled curiosity and much greater capacity than you had dreamed possible.

And do it

One Step at a Time, the final journey can be one of the best.

This Book Wouldn't Have Been Written Without These Folks

I would not have written this book were it not for my wife, **Joyce Jensen**, who's nudged me at critical moments. She ever-so-gently urges me to keep on at whatever, whether it was to finish writing the book or just getting out the door on my daily hike when I'm dragging aimlessly about the house. Joy would rather I end my days on a trail doing what I enjoy most than in a wheelchair at some assisted living home.

And I'd not want to miss thanking my daughter, **Katie Kemsley**, for being first to urge me to write an inspirational hiking book for boomers-becoming-geezers. "Dad, you've taught me so much about hiking. A lot of older people would like to hear why you've kept on hiking all your years."

And, if it weren't for my hiking partner, **Erik Steinberg**, I'd very likely already be in a wheelchair! What a gift of Providence for me to meet Erik shortly after he retired to New Mexico a few years ago. We immediately began hiking together once or twice a week. Shortly thereafter, I had a disabling sciatic attack that had me home-bound and unable to walk across a room. Even on crutches! Erik teamed up with my wife. They insisted I get back onto the trails and do whatever little I could each day. At first, just barely able to get out of the car and waddle to the trailhead and back. Then gradually just a few steps further each day until I was actually stretching those steps into about fifty yards or so. Then to a quarter of a mile. One yard-by-yard creeping up to a half-mile. Until finally walking the entire mile-long loop trail.

Meantime, Erik showed me trick after trick to fix my hiking and eliminate more of the pain. And I did push through still one more day on the trail, regardless of how few steps I might take. Each day, with just a puny number of steps, turned into a triumph!

While not a direct help with the book, there have been so many fine hiking partners who've taught me little tricks, which over the years, have enhanced my love of hearing my boots crunch the grit of the trails. Among the dozens most endearing and enduring was my most frequent partner ever, my nephew **Kenn Petsch**. He doesn't even realize how so many of his trail idiosyncrasies have crept into my own personal trail habits enriching my love of the outdoors, especially the Southwest deserts and Our Favorite, the mighty Grand Canyon.

And there were my ranger heroes with whom I've trod "secret" trails. **Steve Bridgehouse** stands out for his showing Kenn and me many hidden nooks of the Grand Canyon, and eventually his stewardship as Superintendent of a National Monument in Utah.

For the most in-depth wilderness backpack I've ever experienced I owe inexpressible gratitude to USFS's **Bill Holman**. He took me on an extended trek into the heart of the Selway-Bitterroot Wilderness in Idaho. Holman had been super of the Bitterroot National Forest for a number of years before he was assigned to office duties in DC. So, he knew this wilderness intimately. In the 1970s when *Backpacker* was still a fledgling magazine, Bill invited me to see some of the different types of issues the Forest Service had in managing wilderness compared to their usual type of forest management.

USFS's **Bill Wurf** came to give me greater sensitivity to wilderness issues. Wurf was a key author in drafting the 1964 Wilderness Act. And we were out in this prize wilderness forest just a little over a decade later. I did, of course, become quite well-informed about wilderness issues. But, more important, I had a splendid backcountry time with two of the most intense wilderness enthusiasts I'd ever met. Their backcountry camping style was so familiar it was if we'd always known each other. We had fresh-caught trout fried for breakfast at a primitive camp next to an alpine lake. As we hiked, Wurf introduced me to at least a half dozen different blueberry species. We struggled through thick woodland blow-downs on intentionally un-maintained trail deep in the Selway-Bitterroot Wilderness. We joked and fussed as if we'd been together dozens of years; immersed ourselves in the secret depths of nature in its most primitive state; we honestly regretted parting company at the end of our week-long trek.

They stand out among the myriad rangers with whom I've hiked and was blessed to befriend over the years, though today I am fortunate to have such local ranger friends as **Paul Schilke** who dubbed me "Backpacker Bill."

And my ranger hero of what I believe the poster of a ranger ought to be, my buddy **Craig Saum**. With huge crosscut saw on his shoulder, Craig has a whole-hearted devotion to keeping the 600-miles of trails in his jurisdiction cleared for use, each mile of them.

Then, golly, how to thank a hiking partner who has done so much for long trails, my longest-time friend, **Jim Kern**, who takes it in stride for having founded the Florida Trail, co-founded the American Hiking Society and numerous other very important organizations. Jim and I have had so many great adventures in the back woods in so many places, it's hard to keep track. Though one of the most memorable was bushwhacking in the Catskill Mountains seeking a remote location in the headwaters of a creek where our hero, John Burroughs, had caught his prized trout.

And too, our late friend, **Gudy Gaskill**, founder of the Colorado Trail section of the Continental Divide Trail, was a very tough lady to follow on a December backpacking jaunt from eighteen inches of snow on the rim, a few days down along the Tonto Plateau.

Should I leave out my old friend, **Justus Bauschinger**, who had such confidence in the idea of a backpacking magazine that he took the outside back cover from the first issue and became a real personal friend ever after. He'd be right up front in line of supporters for my writing this too, if I asked.

Then, too, how dare I leave out my youngest brother, **Michael Kemsley**, who was on a few, and amazingly best backpacking trips with me in Paraia Canyon, the Grand Canyon, Baxter, Maine and most recently my last and most enjoyable backpacking trip of all, the Rio Grande Gorge here in New Mexico. We hike together as compatible as brothers can be!

Then, would it be fair not to mention **Steve Ifill**, who conducted me on a rare rehabilitation hike through the hallways of the Raymond G. Murphy Veterans Memorial Hospital in Albuquerque to keep my legs limber during one of my confinements in the Cardiac Unit.

I would be greatly remiss not to thank my dear old friend, **Lou Perez**, for his good company on so many of the group treks I organized in various back country meccas as the Bob Marshall Wilderness, the Grand Canyon and the Elk Range in Colorado. The excuse for Lou to be on these excursions was as our "trip physician." But of course! Truth be told, though, it was because Lou was one of my all-time favorite friends.

My pen is running short of ink. I'm sure that my 93-year-old memory has major gaps of others who I owe deepest gratitude for all the back woods knowledge I've gathered from the many miles of trails I've trod with you.

So sorry if I've missed you.

Already, before I put my pen down (I really do write longhand with pen and paper), **Laura Waterman**, my magazine's first editor, comes to mind, and her husband, **Guy Waterman**. We did some amazing hikes together. On one of them, Laura climbed the last winter peak of the 4000-Footers Club list in the Adirondacks of New York. I didn't realize I was suffering a collapsed lung. And I fell asleep for about thirty-six hours in the mountain lean-to while she was off picking off that last peak on her list with her husband, Guy.

Thanks to all of you as well as to others I am sure to have neglected. Especially of course, to my friend, **Larry Luxenberg**, and editor, **George Blackburn**, and book designer, **Alan Strackeljahn**, for their patience with cranky old backpacker Bill, and for Larry's persistence in bringing this book quickly to press, I owe special thanks for his willingness to put up with my picayune geezering.

William Kemsley Jr.
Sept. 9, 2021
Taos, New Mexico

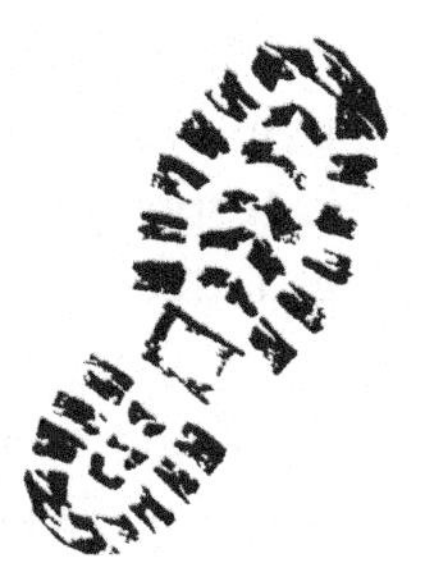

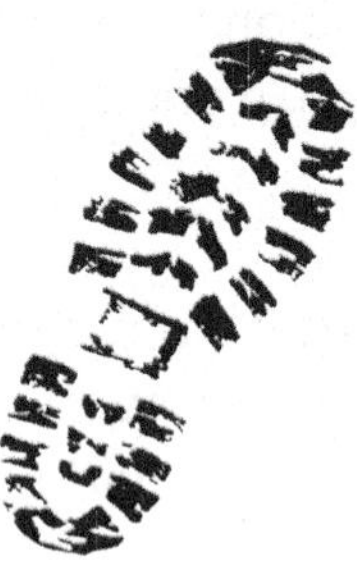

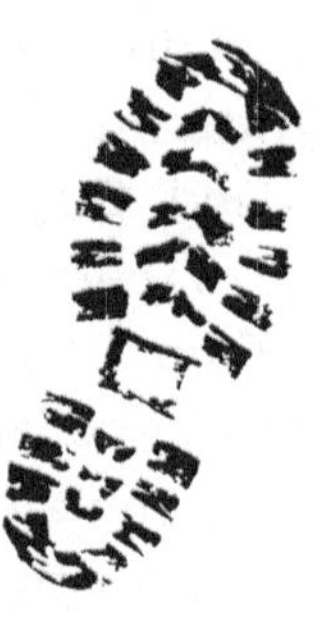

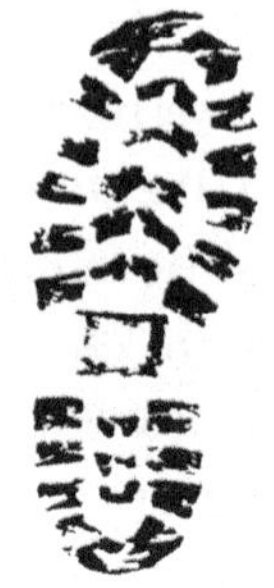

Made in the USA
Monee, IL
03 November 2021

81054298R00075